Immune Response Activation and Immunomodulation

Edited by Rajeev K. Tyagi and Prakash S. Bisen

Published in London, United Kingdom

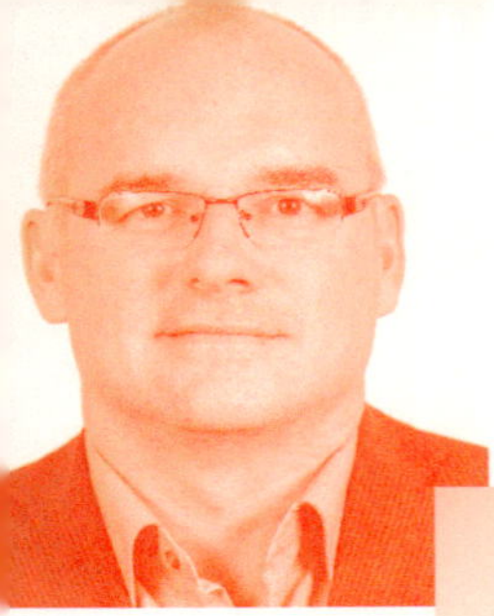
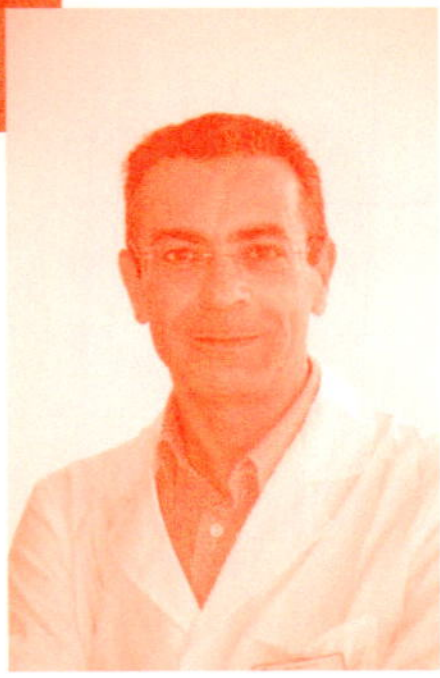
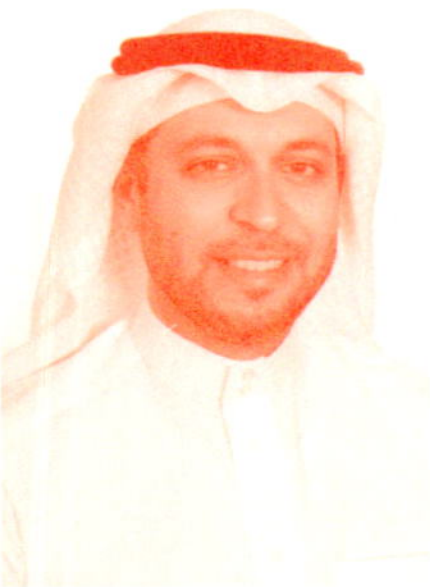
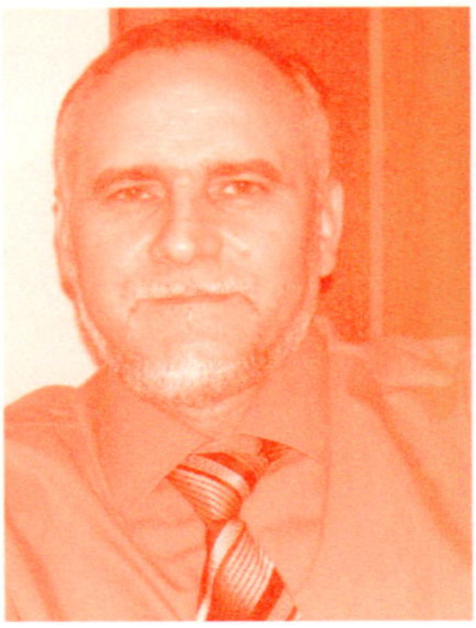
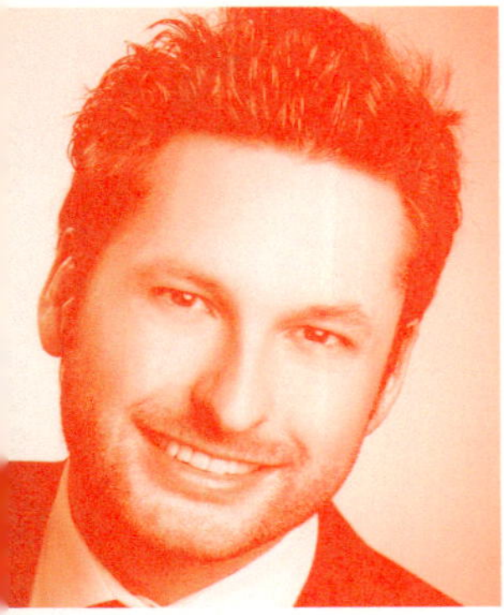
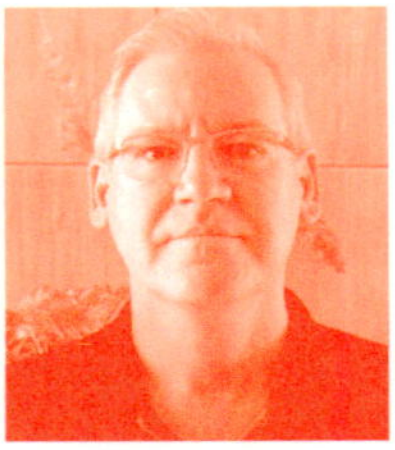
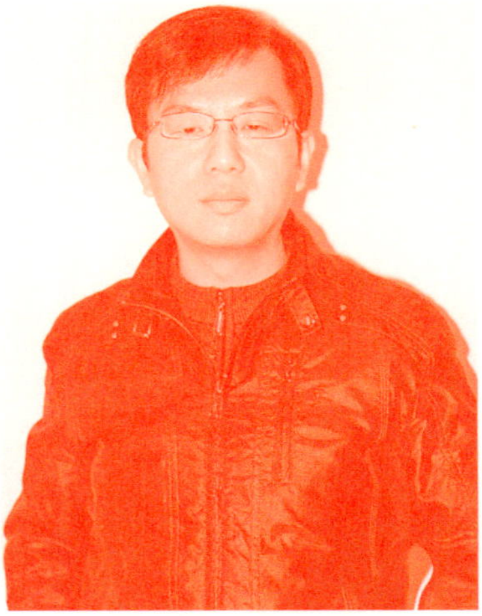

IntechOpen

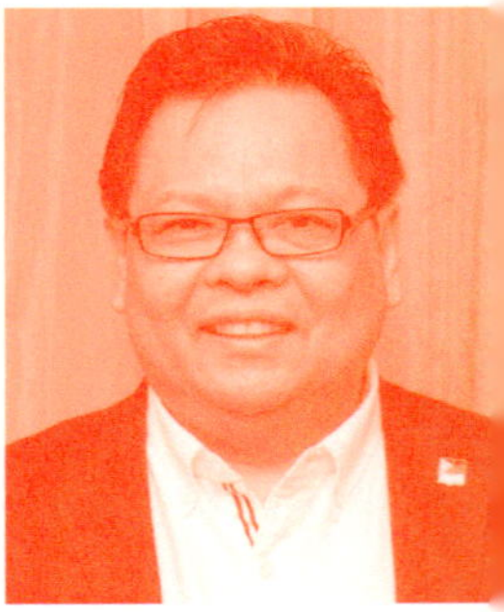
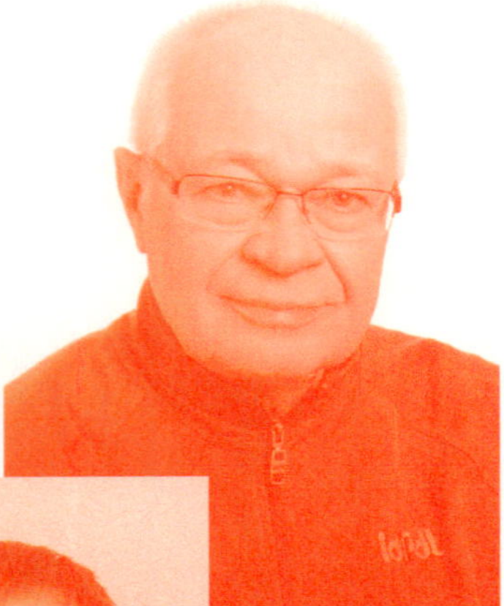
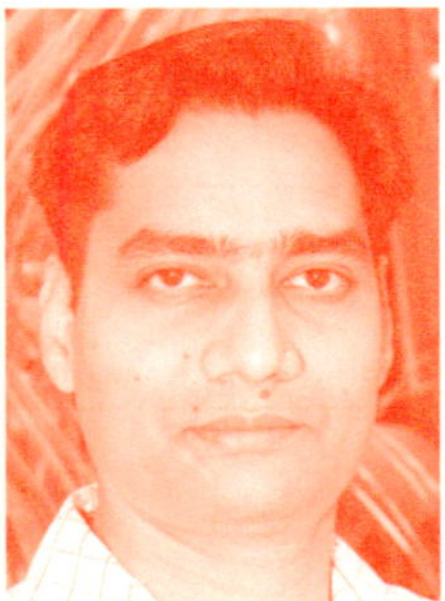
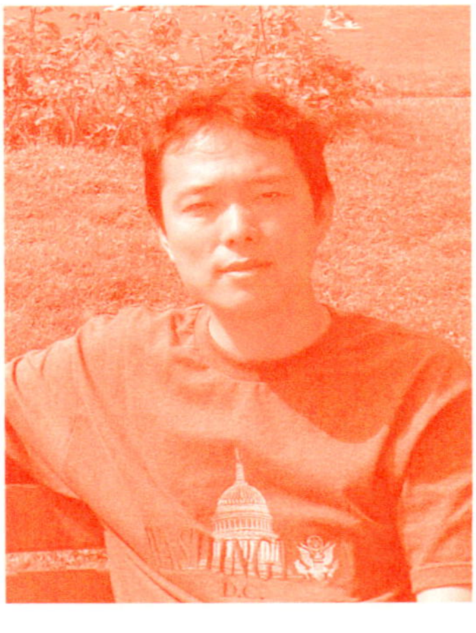
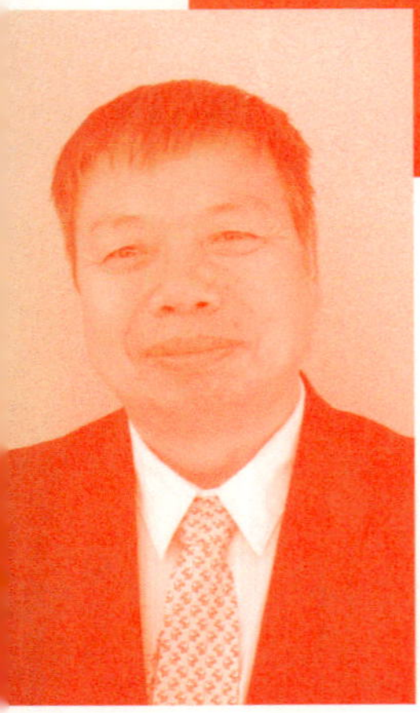
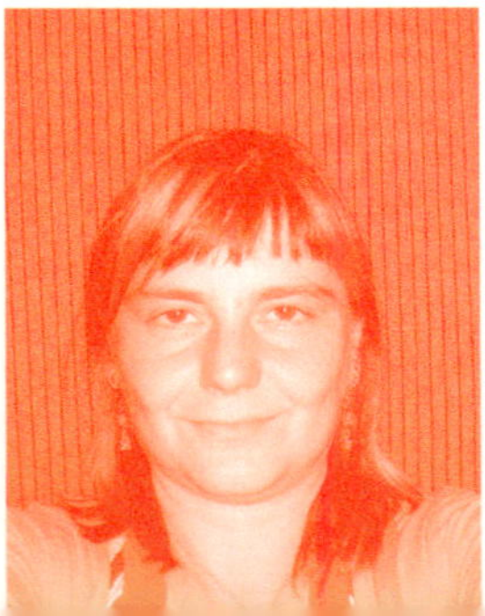

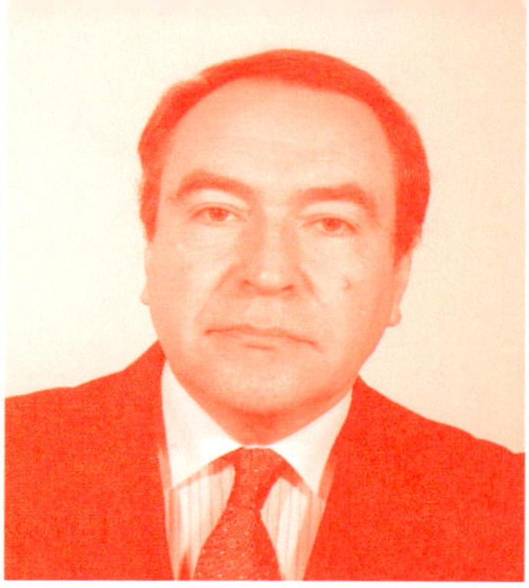
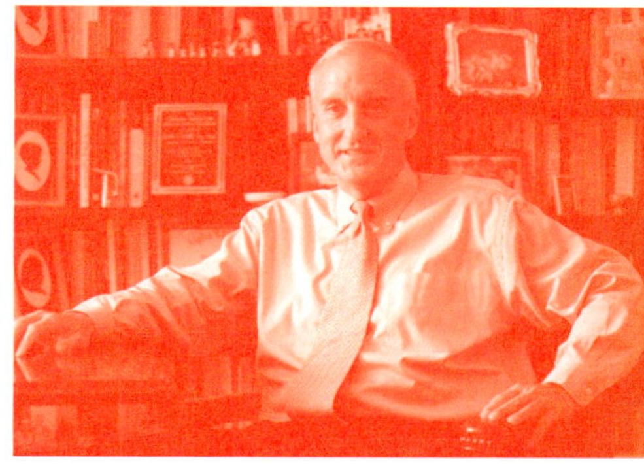
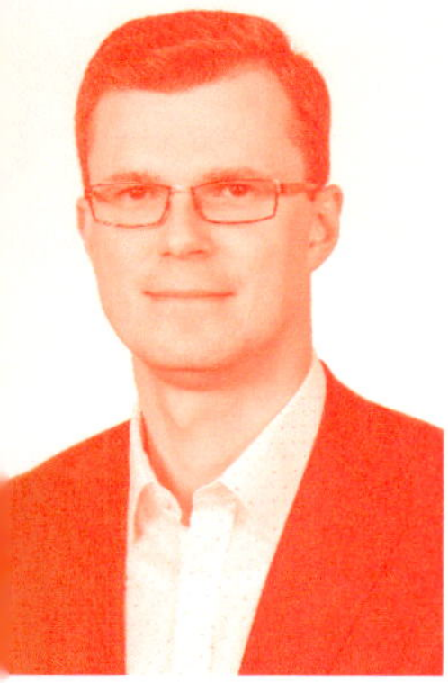
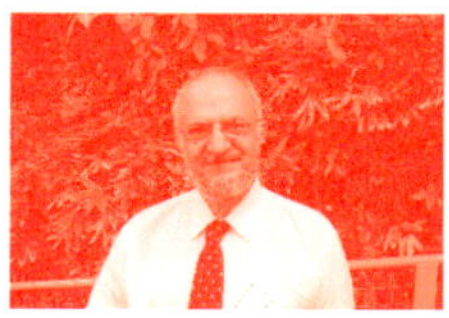
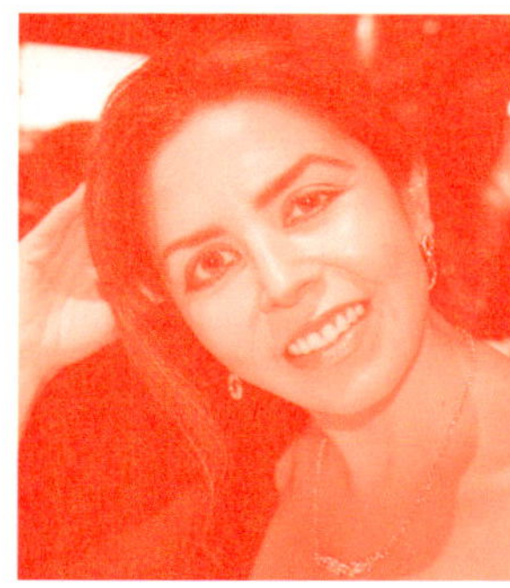

Supporting open minds since 2005

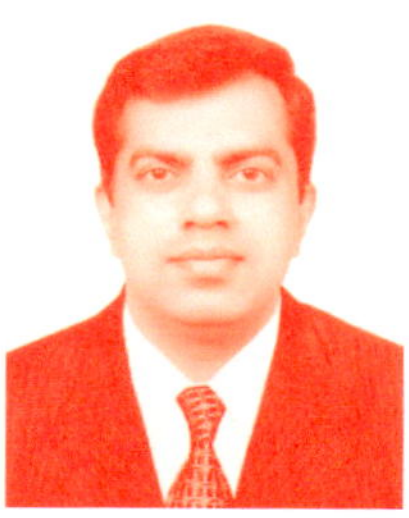
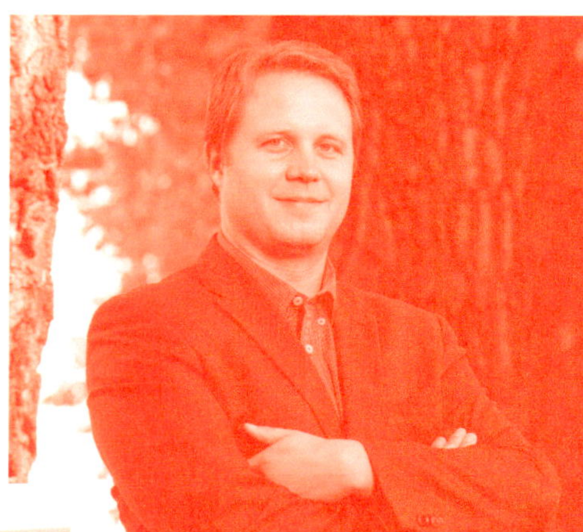
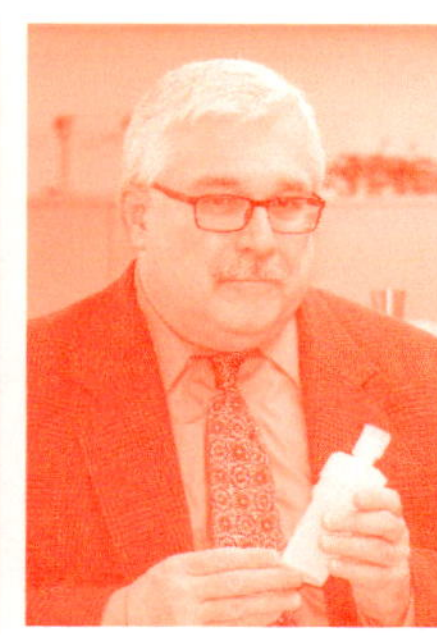
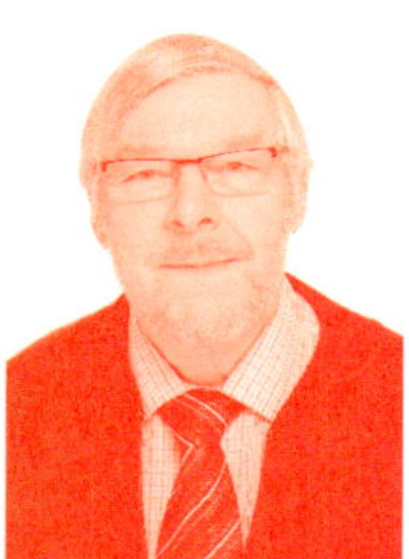
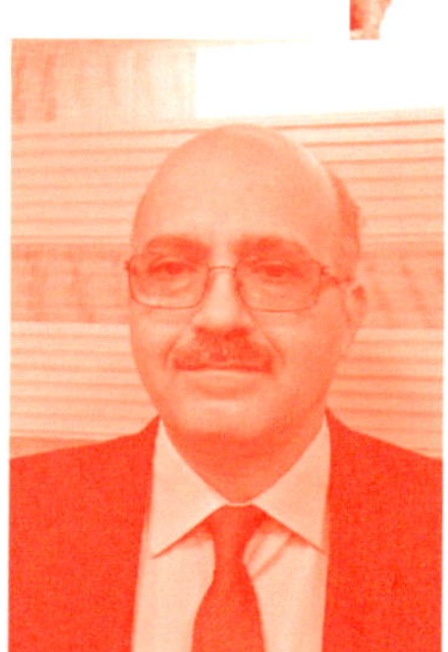
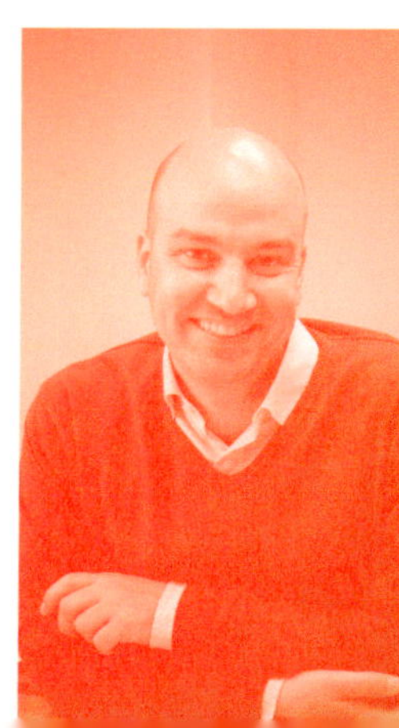
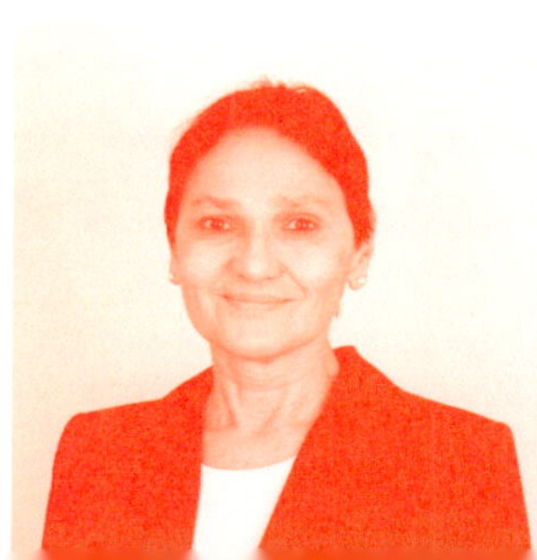

Immune Response Activation and Immunomodulation
http://dx.doi.org/10.5772/intechopen.73708
Edited by Rajeev K. Tyagi and Prakash S. Bisen

Contributors
Dr. Hana'A Burezq, Jose Luis Muñoz-Carrillo, Juan Francisco Contreras Cordero, Oscar Gutiérrez-Coronado, Paola Trinidad Villalobos-Gutiérrez, Viridiana Elizabeth Hernández-Reyes, Luis Guillermo Ramos-Gracia, Maria Del Mar Ortega-Villaizan, Veronica Chico, Sara Puente-Marin, Ivan Nombela, Sultan Gulce Iz, Pelin Saglam Metiner, Sujata Mohanty, Sonali Rawat, Suchi Gupta, Suman Kapur, Dora Patricia Rosete, Carlos Cabello-Gutierrez, Rajeev K. Tyagi

First published in London, United Kingdom, 2019 by IntechOpen
IntechOpen is the global imprint of INTECHOPEN LIMITED, registered in England and Wales, registration number: 11086078, The Shard, 25th floor, 32 London Bridge Street
London, SE19SG – United Kingdom
Printed in Croatia

British Library Cataloguing-in-Publication Data
A catalogue record for this book is available from the British Library

Additional hard copies can be obtained from orders@intechopen.com

Immune Response Activation and Immunomodulation
Edited by Rajeev K. Tyagi and Prakash S. Bisen
p. cm.
Print ISBN 978-1-78985-151-9
Online ISBN 978-1-78985-152-6

For EU product safety concerns:
IN TECH d.o.o., Prolaz Marije Krucifikse Kozulić 3, 51000 Rijeka, Croatia, info@intechopen.com or visit our website at intechopen.com.

Meet the editors

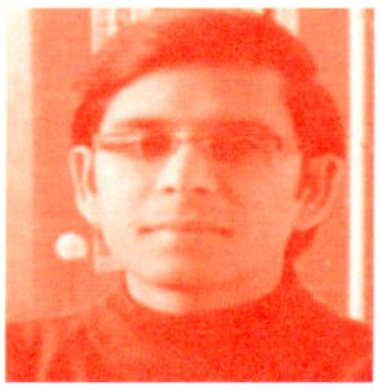

Dr. Rajeev K. Tyagi completed his master's degree in biotechnology at Meerut University, India. Dr. Tyagi completed his doctorate (PhD) in immunology/parasitology/infectiology with a special mention of "*Tres Honorable*" at the Biomedical Parasitology Unit, Institute Pasteur, Paris, France (2011), on a very challenging and demanding area of translational biomedical research. He developed "humanized" mouse model(s) to study asexual blood- and liver-stage infection of *Plasmodium falciparum*. Dr. Tyagi worked at the University of South Florida as a postdoc fellow, and he used the developed humanized mouse to characterize the attenuated asexual blood-stage *falciparum* parasite as well as made efforts to develop human-liver chimeric mice using TK/NOG mice to study liver-stage infections of *P. falciparum*. Dr. Tyagi deployed his efforts to understand pathogen-differentiated dendritic cells and their implications in developing therapeutic interventional approaches for chronic periodontitis and other systemic inflammatory disorders during his second postdoc at Augusta University. Dr. Tyagi has been making efforts to understand the role of nanocarriers to develop therapeutic approaches to address cancer and systemic inflammatory diseases. Currently, Dr. Tyagi is working as a research scientist at Vanderbilt University Medical Center, Nashville, USA, trying to understand and develop interventional approaches against colitis.

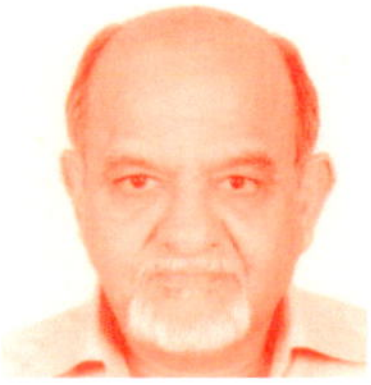

Prof. Prakash Singh Bisen earned his PhD in 1972 and was awarded a DSc in 1981. After his postdoctoral work, he worked as an assistant professor at Jabalpur University where he was promoted to associate professor. He then joined Bhopal University as a professor of microbiology in 1985. Prof. Bisen was a visiting professor at the Institute of Environmental and Biological Sciences, University of Lancaster, England, and the Department of Biological Sciences, University of Illinois at Chicago. He was a US National Science Foundation Fellow at the University of California at Davis and Berkeley working in the Department of Bacteriology on DNA recombinant technology. Prof. Bisen was a WHO/UNESCO Fellow for one year at the Institute of Microbiology, Czechoslovak Academy of Sciences, Budejovika, Praha, Czechoslovakia, and UNESCO/UNDP/ICRO and Hungarian Academy of Sciences Fellow at the Institute of Plant Physiology, Biological Research Center, Szeged, Hungary. He is honored with a Life Time Professorship at Bundelkhand University, Jhansi, India, the highest award of the university. He worked as the emeritus scientist (CSIBerkeleyR) at the Defence Research Development Establishment, Defence Research Development Organization, Ministry of Defence, Government of India, Gwalior, India, and is presently an honorary professor of biotechnology at Jiwaji University. Prof. Bisen guided 65 doctoral theses and has 300 publications to his credit. He has published six international patents in the United States, Europe, Japan, and India. He has been awarded 6 international patents and 12 are under consideration.

Contents

Preface

This book is an effort to reflect on the new advances in our understanding of the immune system, immune response activation, as well as immunomodulation, and to improve upon the presentation of information to students, teachers, and researchers. As teachers of immunology, we are becoming increasingly aware that assimilating detailed information as well as experimental approaches is difficult in many medical school and undergraduate courses. The problem of how much detail is appropriate has become a pressing issue because of the continuous and rapid increase in the amount of information in biomedical sciences. This problem is compounded by the development of integrated curricula in many medical schools, with reduced time for didactic teaching and an increasing emphasis on social and behavioural sciences and primary health. For all these reasons, we have realized the value for many medical students of presenting the principles of immunology in a concise and clear manner.

This book has been written to address the perceived needs of both medical school and undergraduate curricula and to take advantage of new understandings in immunology. We have tried to achieve several goals and present the most important principles governing the function of the immune system. Our fundamental objective has been to synthesize the key concepts from the vast amount of experimental data that have emerged in the rapidly advancing field of immunology. The choice of what is most important is based on what is most clearly established by experimentation, what our students find puzzling, and what explains the wonderful efficiency and economy of the immune system. Inevitably, however, such a choice will have an element of bias, and our bias is toward emphasizing the cellular interactions in the immune response by limiting the description of many of the underlying biochemical and molecular mechanisms to the essential facts. This book gives an insight into the role of cytokines in activating immune response during a pathogenic invasion. Immunomodulation, aryl hydrocarbons, the role of the protein defensin and nucleated cells in provoking the immune response, Bcl protein/gene-based apoptotic pathways, and plant-derived phytochemical-mediated immune response are all central themes of the book.

In essence, I very strongly believe that the content of this book will be helpful to those working on the immunology of infectious diseases and beyond.

Rajeev K. Tyagi, PhD
Department of Medicine,
Division of Gastroenterology,
Hepatology and Nutrition Vanderbilt University Medical Centre (VUMC),
Nashville, USA

Prakash S. Bisen, PhD
Honorary Emeritus Professor,
School of Studies in Biotechnology,
Jiwaji University,
Gwalior, MP, India

Section 1

Immune Response Activation

Chapter 1

Introductory Chapter: Immunity and Immunomodulation

Rajeev K. Tyagi

1. Introduction

The mammalian immune system is comprised of two branches of immune system; innate and adaptive, which render tolerance towards host for protection from microbial infections. The innate immune system consists of functionally distinct mechanism that evolved to render protection against pathogens. The nonadaptive immune system senses pathogens through pattern recognition receptors which trigger the activation of antimicrobial defense system to stimulate and provoke the efficient immune response. The acquired immune system in response activates the nonadaptive immune effector mechanisms in an antigen-specific and dependent manner. Although the link between various immune components are not fully understood, recent progresses bring us closer to an integrated view of immune system and its function towards the host defense [1].

The infectious diseases are the leading cause for the greater rate of morbidity and mortality world-wide and are a major challenge for the biomedical sciences. The physical methods such as improved sanitary conditions, clean water supplies and vector control are by far the most effective measures, development of vaccines and therapeutics are panacea for their treatment. The development of vaccine and therapeutic interventions require the understanding of host immune system. Recently, significant progress has been made towards unraveling the mechanisms of microbial pathogenesis and host-microbe symbiosis. There are many challenges remain and most daunting is the development of effective vaccine. Indeed, it is not known how to elicit protective immunity against most pathogens in a safe and practical manner. To address and overcome the autoimmune response mounted by the host are required and to be explored by the basic science researchers.

The innate immune system is the phylogenically oldest component of the human immune system. The innate immune system is highly complex and consists of barriers to infection (epithelia of skin, gastrointestinal, respiratory, genitourinary tracts), antimicrobial peptides and proteins, humoral components (i.e., complement and opsonins) and cellular components (i.e., neutrophils, monocytes/macrophages, dendritic cells, and innate lymphoid cells). Innate immunity serves as the front line of host defense and plays an essential role in preventing infection while tolerating normal host flora. The defects in innate immunity are associated with invasive, life-threatening infection, and inappropriate activation of innate immune system may lead to auto-inflammatory states. The innate immune system directs the subsequent development of adaptive immune responses [2].

The human acquired immune system is responsible for the destruction of foreign particles once they have entered the body. During the first exposure to an invader (which could be a virus, a bacteria or any unwanted particle), the acquired immune system must "learn" how to attack and destroy the foreign particle. This implies that adaptive system is not as active and efficient in the clearance of any pathogens as innate immune system [3].

Activation of acquired immune system: unlike the innate immune system, the acquired immune system needs to be exposed with a substance before its effective action. The acquired immune system is target specific and takes its own time to prepare to act against pathogens [3].

1.1 Role of cytokines in the immune response activation and immunomodulation

Cytokines participate in many physiological processes including the regulation of immune and inflammatory responses. These effector molecules are produced transiently and locally and control the quantum of amplitude and duration of the response. The research outcomes have shown that meagre or suboptimal production of these informational molecules may significantly contribute to the pathophysiology of various diseases [4]. Particularly the cytokines released by $CD4^+$ T cells at the onset of an immune response are decisive for pathological or physiological consequences. IL-1, IL-4, IL-6, IL-10, IL-12, TNF-alpha and IFN-alpha, -beta, -gamma, etc., are known to contribute to the pathophysiology of autoimmune diseases, infectious diseases, and allograft rejection [4].

The inflammatory responses in the peripheral and central nervous systems play key roles in the development and persistence of many pathological pain states [5]. Cytokine a broader name which includes lymphokine; cytokines secreted by the lymphocytes, monokines are secreted by the cells of myeloid origin such as monocytes, chemokine shows chemotactic activities, and the interleukins are the cytokines made by one leukocyte which acts on other leukocytes. The cytokines may act on the cells that secrete them in an autocrine manner or on nearby cells following the paracrine fashion. The action in some instances on distant cells is termed as "endocrine action" [6].

1.2 Pro-inflammatory cytokines

An inflammatory or pro-inflammatory cytokine is a type of signaling molecule that is excreted by the cells of immune cells such as helper T cells (Th) and macrophages, and some other cell types which are known to promote inflammation as a defense mechanism. The interleukin-1 (IL-1), IL-12, and IL-18, tumor necrosis factor (TNF), interferon gamma (IFN-γ), and granulocyte-macrophage colony stimulating (GM-CSF) factor and play an important role in mediating and regulating the nonadaptive immune response. The inflammatory cytokines are predominantly produced by and involved in the upregulation of inflammatory reactions to show resistance towards infectious pathogen [7, 8].

1.3 Anti-inflammatory cytokines

The anti-inflammatory cytokines are a series of immunoregulatory molecules that control pro-inflammatory cytokines, production and their response. The cytokines act in concert with specific cytokine inhibitors and soluble cytokine receptors with an objective to regulate the human immune response. Their physiologic role in provoking inflammatory responses and pathologic role in systemic inflammatory states are increasingly recognized. The chief anti-inflammatory cytokines include interleukin (IL)-1 receptor antagonist, IL-4, IL-6, IL-10, IL-11, and IL-13. The specific cytokine receptors for IL-1, tumor necrosis factor-α and IL-18 also function as the inhibitors of the pro-inflammatory cytokines [9, 10].

1.4 Immunomodulation

Mesenchymal Stem Cells (MSCs) emerging as key players in regenerative medicine for the treatment of various inflammatory and infectious diseases. The MSCs are emerging an effective tool in developing therapeutic interventional approaches and further advancements. Several tissues have been identified as potential sources of MSCs including bone marrow, cord blood, dental pulp, umbilical cord, adipose tissue, peripheral blood, fetal liver, of which some are clinically recognized. MSCs activate the immune responses and inhibit proliferation, maturation and differentiation of T and B cells. The MSCs activated immune response induce the expression of regulatory T cells (Tregs) [11] which are very important in regulating the immune system and immune effecters of diseased cells.

The immune response activation and immunomodulation is an essential reading to all medical students, biologist, biochemist, and professionals involved in the field of immunology of infectious diseases and beyond. The book is a useful and ideal guide for novice researchers interested in learning research methods to unravel the knot of immune responses and their activation. The role of various cytokines in mounting the protective/immune response as well as during immunomodulation is the central theme of this book.

Author details

Rajeev K. Tyagi
Department of Medicine, Division of Gastroenterology, Hepatology and Nutrition, Vanderbilt University Medical Centre (VUMC), Nashville, TN, USA

*Address all correspondence to: rajeev.tyagi@vumc.org; rajeev.dbt@gmail.com

References

[1] Medzhitov R. Recognition of microorganisms and activation of the immune response. Nature. 2007;**449**:819-826

[2] Shishido SN, Varahan S, Yuan K, Li X, Fleming SD. Humoral innate immune response and disease. Clinical Immunology. 2012;**144**:142-158

[3] Chaplin DD. Overview of the immune response. The Journal of Allergy and Clinical Immunology. 2010;**125**:S3-S23

[4] Van der Meide PH, Schellekens H. Cytokines and the immune response. Biotherapy. 1996;**8**:243-249

[5] Watkins LR, Milligan ED, Maier SF. Glial proinflammatory cytokines mediate exaggerated pain states: Implications for clinical pain. Advances in Experimental Medicine and Biology. 2003;**521**:1-21

[6] Wen H, Gao Y, An JY, Chen QL, Zheng JP. Evaluation of exercise intensity for pulmonary rehabilitation in patients with chronic obstructive pulmonary disease. Zhonghua Jie He He Hu Xi Za Zhi. 2007;**30**:27-30

[7] Cavaillon JM. Pro- versus anti-inflammatory cytokines: Myth or reality. Cellular and Molecular Biology (Noisy-le-Grand, France). 2001;**47**:695-702

[8] Zhang JM, An J. Cytokines, inflammation, and pain. International Anesthesiology Clinics. 2007;**45**:27-37

[9] Opal SM, DePalo VA. Anti-inflammatory cytokines. Chest. 2000;**117**:1162-1172

[10] Arango Duque G, Descoteaux A. Macrophage cytokines: Involvement in immunity and infectious diseases. Frontiers in Immunology. 2014;**5**:491

[11] Cagliani J, Grande D, Molmenti EP, Miller EJ, Rilo HLR. Immunomodulation by mesenchymal stromal cells and their clinical applications. Journal of Stem Cell and Regenerative Biology. 2017;**3**(2). DOI: 10.15436/2471-0598.17.022. PMID: 29104965

Section 2

Role of Cytokines in Immune System Activation

Chapter 2

Cytokine Profiling Plays a Crucial Role in Activating Immune System to Clear Infectious Pathogens

José Luis Muñoz-Carrillo, Juan Francisco Contreras-Cordero, Oscar Gutiérrez-Coronado, Paola Trinidad Villalobos-Gutiérrez, Luis Guillermo Ramos-Gracia and Viridiana Elizabeth Hernández-Reyes

Abstract

Pathogen infections are recognized by the immune system, which consists of two types of responses: an innate immune response that recognizes pathogen-associated molecular patterns (PAMPs) and an antigen-specific adaptive immune response. In both responses, there are several activated cells of the immune system, which play a key role in establishing the environment of cytokines, thus directing their differentiation either suppressing or promoting the immune response. This immune response is crucial against pathogen infections. In this chapter, we will describe the crucial role played by different families of cytokines during activation of the immune system to eliminate infectious pathogens.

Keywords: cytokines, IL-1, TNF, IL-17, IL-6, IFN, bacteria, fungi, virus, parasites

1. Introduction

The innate and adaptive immune responses are key factors in the control of infections or chronic diseases. The balance between these two systems is mainly orchestrated by cytokines [1]. Cytokines are low-molecular-weight proteins that contribute to the chemical language that regulates the development and repair of tissues, hematopoiesis, inflammation, etc., through the transduction of signals mediated by binding to cellular receptors. Cytokines can act on their target cells in an autocrine, paracrine, and/or endocrine fashion to induce systemic and/or localized immune responses. In addition, cytokines have pleiotropic activity, that is, they act on different target cells, as well as affect the function of other cytokines in an additive, synergistic, or antagonistic manner [2, 3]. Cytokines can be secreted by immune cells, but they can also be produced by a wide variety of cells in response to infection or can be produced or released from cells in response to cellular damage when cellular integrity is compromised. Acting through a series of conserved signaling pathways that program transcriptional pathways by controlling many biological processes, such as cell growth, cell differentiation, apoptosis, development, and survival, can also reprogram cells in the local tissue environment to improve certain types of immune responses. Therefore, cytokines are critical mediators of communication for the immune system and are essential for host defense against pathogens [4].

2. Cytokines

The cytokine pattern that is released from the cell depends primarily on the nature of the antigenic stimulus and the type of cell being stimulated. Cytokines compromise leukocytes to respond to a microbial stimulus. Cytokines can be classified into six groups: (1) L1 superfamily, (2) TNF superfamily, (3) IL-17 family, (4) IL-6 superfamily, (5) type I superfamily, and (6) type II superfamily [5].

2.1 IL-1 superfamily

More than any other cytokine family, the interleukin (IL)-1 family of ligands and receptors is primarily associated with acute and chronic inflammation. The cytosolic segment of each IL-1 receptor family member contains the Toll/interleukin-1 receptor (TIR) domain. This domain is also present in each Toll-like receptor (TLR), which responds to microbial products and viruses [6]. Since TIR domains are functional for both receptor families, responses to the IL-1 family are fundamental to the innate immunity [7].

2.1.1 IL-1 family of cytokines and innate immune system

There are 11 members of IL-1 family of cytokines (IL-1α, IL-1β, IL-1Ra, IL-18, IL-33, IL-36α, IL-36β, IL-36γ, IL-36Ra IL-37, and IL-38) and 10 members of the IL-1 family of receptors (IL-1R1 to ILR10) [8, 9]. More than any other cytokine family, the IL-1 family members are closely linked to damaging inflammation; however, the same members also work to increase nonspecific resistance to infection and the development of an immune response to a foreign antigen [10].

The numerous biological properties of the IL-1 family are nonspecific. The importance of IL-1 family members to the innate response became evident upon the discovery that the cytoplasmic domain of the IL-1 receptor type 1 (IL-1R1) is also found in the Toll protein of the fruit fly. The functional domain of the cytoplasmic component of IL-1R1 is termed the TIR domain. Thus, fundamental inflammatory responses such as the induction of cyclooxygenase type 2 (COX-2), production of multiple cytokines and chemokines, increased the expression of adhesion molecules, or synthesis of nitric oxide (NO) are indistinguishable responses of both IL-1 and TLR ligands [11]. Both TLR and IL-1 families nonspecifically augment antigen recognition and activate lymphocyte function. The lymphocyte-activating function of IL-1 was first described in 1979 and is now considered a fundamental property of the acquired immune response. IL-1β is the most studied member of the IL-1 family due to its role in mediating auto-inflammatory diseases. Unquestionably, IL-1β evolved to assist host defense against infection, and this landmark study established how a low dose of recombinant IL-1β protects mice against lethal bacterial infection in the absence of neutrophils. Although we now accept the concept that cytokines like IL-1β served millions of years of evolution to protect the host, in the antibiotic and antiviral therapies era of today, we view cytokines as the cause of disease due to acute or chronic inflammation [12]. IL-1β has emerged as a therapeutic target for an expanding number of systemic and local inflammatory conditions called auto-inflammatory diseases. The neutralization of IL-1β results in a rapid and sustained reduction in disease severity. Treatment for autoimmune diseases often includes immunosuppressive drugs, whereas neutralization of IL-1β is mostly anti-inflammatory. The auto-inflammatory diseases are caused due to gain-of-function mutations for caspase-1 activity, and common ailments, such as gout, type 2 diabetes, heart failure, recurrent pericarditis, rheumatoid arthritis, and smoldering myeloma, respond to the IL-1β neutralization [7]. IL-1 family also includes member that suppress inflammation, specifically within the IL-1 family, such as the IL-1 receptor antagonist (IL-1Ra), IL-36 receptor antagonist (IL-36Ra), and IL-37. In addition, the IL-1 family member IL-38, the last member of the IL-1 family of cytokines to be studied, nonspecifically suppresses inflammation and limits the innate immunity [12].

2.1.2 IL-1 receptor family

There are 10 members of the IL-1 family receptors. IL-1R1 binds IL-1α, IL-1β, and IL-1Ra and IL-R1 binds either IL-1β or IL-1α. IL-1R2 is a decoy receptor for IL-1β. IL-1R2 lacks a cytoplasmic domain and exists not only as an integral membrane protein but also in a soluble form. The term soluble is meant to denote the extracellular domain only. The soluble domain of IL-1R2 binds IL-1β in the extracellular space and neutralizes IL-1β. The neutralization of IL-1β by soluble IL-1R2 is greatly enhanced by forming a complex with IL-1R3. IL-1R3 is the co-receptor for IL-1α, IL-1β, IL-33, IL-36a, IL-36β, and IL-36γ. IL-1R3 exists as an integral membrane receptor or in a soluble receptor form. The inflammation and infection drive liver to increase the synthesis and levels of soluble IL-1R3 in the circulation [13].

2.2 TNF superfamily

Tumor necrosis factor superfamily (TNFSF) is a group of cytokines composed of 19 ligands and 29 receptors [14]. This family plays a pivotal role in immunity, inflammation and controlling cell cycle, proliferation, differentiation, and apoptosis [15]. TNFSF receptors can be divided into two different groups depending on the presence or absence of the intracellular death domain (DD) [16]. Signaling via the death domain demands the involvement of adapter proteins Fas-associated death domain (FADD) and TNF receptor-associated proteins (TRADD), leading to the activation of caspases that result in apoptotic death of a cell. The second group of TNFSF receptor signals acts only via adapter proteins termed tumor necrosis factor receptor-associated proteins (TRAFs). The DD containing receptors may use the pathway [17]. The functional activity of TNFSF receptors depends on the cellular context and the balance between pro- and antiapoptotic factors inside the cell and in the environment. Mostly, the TNFSF members are revealed on the cells of immune system and play a notable function in maintaining the equilibrium of T-cell–mediated immune responses by arranging direct signals required for the full activation of effector pool and survival of memory T cells. The TNFSF members are necessary in the development of pathogenesis of many T-cell–mediated autoimmune diseases, such as asthma, diabetes, and arthritis [16].

2.2.1 TNF-α

Tumor necrosis factor (TNF)-α is classified as homotrimeric transmembrane protein with a prominent role in systemic inflammation. Macrophages/monocytes are capable to produce TNF-α in the acute phase of inflammation, and this cytokine drives a wide range of signaling events within cells, leading to necrosis or apoptosis [17]. The TNF superfamily incorporates receptor activator of nuclear factor κB

(RANK), cluster of differentiation (CD)-40, CD27, and FAS receptor. This protein was discovered in the circulation of animals subsequent to the stimulation of their reticuloendothelial system and lipopolysaccharide (LPS) challenge. This protein has been found to provoke a rapid necrotic regression of certain forms of tumors [16].

2.2.2 Biological roles of TNF-α

Several biological functions are ascribed to the TNF-α, and for this reason, the mechanism of action is somewhat complex. Because this protein confers resistance to certain types of infections and in parallel causes pathological complications, it carries out contradictory roles. This may be connected to the varied signaling pathways that are activated. TNF-α modulates several therapeutic roles within the body, such as immunostimulation, resistance to infection agents, resistance to tumors, sleep regulation, and embryonic development [17]. On the other hand, parasitic, bacterial, and viral infections become more pathogenic or fatal due to TNF circulation. The major role of TNF is explicated as mediator in resistance against infections. Moreover, it was postulated that TNF plays a pathological role in several autoimmune diseases such as graft versus host rejection or rheumatoid arthritis. In addition, TNF exhibits antimalignant cell cytotoxicity in association with interferon. High concentrations of TNF-α are toxic to the host. The enhancement in the therapeutic index by decreasing toxicity or by increasing effectiveness is indeed needed. This may be possible through the mutations that reduce systemic cytotoxicity and increase TNF's effectiveness in selectively eliminating tumor cells. TNF-α is also implicated in physiological sleep regulation. TNF-related proteins such as receptor activator for nuclear factor κB ligand (RANKL) are required for osteoclast differentiation necessary for bone resorption [16].

2.3 IL-17 family

IL-17 is a pro-inflammatory cytokine. There are six family known members of IL-17. Also, we have just a little information of its biological functions, being the IL-17A and the IL-17F described recently [18]. IL-17–related cytokines play key roles in defense against extracellular pathogen, and their participation in the development of autoimmune diseases has drawn significant attention. Moreover, some of these molecules are involved in the amplification and perpetuation of pathological processes in many inflammatory diseases. However, the same cytokines can exert anti-inflammatory effects in specific settings, as well as play a key role in the control of immune homeostasis [19, 20].

2.4 IL-6 superfamily

IL-6 family is a group of cytokines and colony-stimulating factors (CSFs) that include IL-6, IL-27, IL-31, IL-35, ciliary neurotrophic factor (CNTF), leukemia inhibitory factor (LIF), oncostatin M (OSM), cardiotrophin (CT)-1, and cardiotrophin-like cytokine (CLC), among others [16, 17]. This cytokine family binds to its receptor, allowing a binding with the gp130 subunit [21, 22]. This binding allows dimerization of the subunit homogeneously or heterogeneously (either with the same subunit or cytokine receptor), creating a receptor complex. This complex allows associated proteins phosphorylation, such as Janus kinases (JAK) type 1, 2, and tyrosine kinase (TYK) 2, among others, which triggers a signaling pathway through phosphorylation toward types of signal transducer and activator of transcription (STAT) 1–6, forming another dimerization, homogeneous or heterogeneous with other STATs, that gets into the nucleus, recognizing promoter regions and initiating the regulation of the expression of specific genes [22, 23].

In IL-6 family, there are soluble receptors that have different signaling pathways, which are mostly of inhibitory function. Although they bind to the same cytokine and to the same subunit, they transmit different signaling called trans-signaling. It is observed that these soluble receptors prolong its effect and have action on cells where cytokine emerges effect; namely, all cells reactive to IL-6 will have the soluble receptor of IL-6 (IL-6Rs) function [21, 24]. Main functions of this IL-6 family cytokines are inflammation proteins production in acute phase, B cell differentiation into antibody-forming plasma cell, T cell modulator, development of Th17, and hematopoiesis, among other functions [24–26].

2.5 Type I superfamily

Type I cytokine family, also known as hematopoietins, is made up of several types of cytokines, including IL-2, IL-3, IL-4, IL-6, IL-7, IL-9, IL-12, IL-15, IL-21, and granulocyte-macrophage colony-stimulating factor (GM-CSF), among others. This group of cytokines has α, β, and γ chain in common. IL-2, -4, -7, -9, -13, -15, and -21 have in common the γ chain (also known as IL2Rγ or CD132) for activation of JAK1/JAK3 and downstream STAT 1–5. While IL-3, -5, and GM-CSF share the common β chain (CSF2RB/CD131) for activation of the JAK/STAT pathway through interactions with JAK2 [3, 27], α chains do not activate signaling pathways but increase the binding affinity between the cytokine and β and γ subunit [3, 28], helping receptor specificity for gene expression [27]. While the receptor is more complex, there is more affinity of the cytokines of the receptor, which increases the signaling [27, 29]. The specificity of the receptor is conferred by α and β subunit, that in combination with γ subunit provides different stimulations. This means that the same cytokines can have different effects on the cell, depending on the receptor complexity; for example, IL-2 binds to its γ chain receptor (CD132) and β chain (IL-2Rβ), forming an intermediate affinity dimer, or also the binding of α chain (IL-2Rα), generating a high affinity. Phosphorylating tyrosine residues in JAKs, which lead to signaling to STAT5, prolonging and increasing its effect unlike the intermediate affinity [30]. Among the main functions of this cytokine family are the growth and differentiation of precursor leukocytes, as well as being modulators and initiators of the inflammatory response [3, 27].

2.6 Type II superfamily

The type II superfamily is composed of the subfamilies of interferons (IFNs) and IL-10. IFN family has the characteristic of inducing antiviral response in both hematopoietic and structural cells, serving as an essential mediator of cross talk between the immune system and host physiology during viral infections [3, 29]. This family is divided into three types INFs families: types I, II, and III.

Type I IFNs family is mainly composed of IFN-α and -β. IFN-α is expressed in leukocytes and IFN-β in fibroblasts, dendritic, and plasmacytoid cells. These IFNs have signaling pathways through JAK1 and TYK2 to phosphorylate STAT1 and STAT2 [29, 31]. These IFNs have a powerful proinflammatory effect and an antiviral response in immune and nonhematopoietic cells, as well as they can synergize with type II interferon (i.e., IFNγ) to potentiate Th1 lineage commitment by T-helper cells and cytotoxic activity by $CD8^+$ cells [3].

Type II IFNs family is composed only by IFN-γ, which is produced by active $CD4^+$ and $CD8^+$ T cells, NK cells, and macrophages by stimulation of IL-12, IL-18, and TNF-α [3, 29, 32]. IFN-γ has signaling pathways with STAT1 through JAK1 and JAK2 [29]. IFN-γ is mediator of interaction of innate and adaptive immune cells. IFN-γ promotes B-cell differentiation toward plasma cells immunoglobulin (Ig)-G-production. Also, IFN-γ induces phagocytosis through the antimicrobial potential activation on macrophages. IFN-γ increases the expression of major histocompatibility complex (MHC) I and II, molecules in antigen-presenting cells, promotes complement activation, and increases cytotoxic activity of T cells and differentiation Th1 cell differentiation for the clearance of infectious pathogens [3, 32].

Type III INFs family is composed by IFNλ-1 (IL-29), IFNλ-2 (IL-28A), and IFNλ-3 (IL-28B) [3, 29, 32]. IFNλ-1 and -2 regulate IFN expression [3], being structurally and functionally like them by sharing beta chain but with less intensity [32]. IFNλ-3 induces antiviral response in cells through STAT1 and STAT2 [3, 33].

IL-10 is a potent pro-inflammatory cytokine, which is produced by different cells such as monocytes, macrophages, Th2, and Treg cells. The IL-10 performs its functions through the activation of the STAT1, STAT3, PI3K, and p38 mitogen-activated protein kinases (MAPK) pathways. Among its most important functions are the suppression of Th1 cytokines, the classically activated/M1 macrophage inflammatory gene expression, and the presentation of antigen [3].

3. Cytokine profile in bacterial infections

During a bacterial infection in the host, a nonspecific and immediate immune response is initiated to eliminate the pathogen, and this nonspecific response involves the recruitment of neutrophils, macrophages and dendritic cells, complement activation, and cytokine production [34]. This response can inhibit or limit microbial growth but also can cause host damage, and so it is necessary to keep this response under control; to achieve this, the host performs some strategies, including the production of cytokines. These molecules play an important role in intercellular communication and coordinate the innate and adaptive response [35].

In microbial infections, the pattern-recognition receptors (PRRs) recognize several PAMPs [36] such as DNA, double-stranded RNA (dsRNA), single-stranded RNA (ssRNA), and 5′-triphosphate RNA, as well as lipoproteins, surface glycoproteins, membrane components peptidoglycans, lipoteichoic acid (LTA), lipopolysaccharide (LPS), and glycosyl-phosphatidyl-inositol. The recognition of PAMPs by PRRs leads to the activation of NF-κB and/or MAPK [37] to produce several cytokines such as IL-1α, IL-1β, TNFα, IFN-γ, IL-12, and IL-18, being TNF-α and IL-1β the main inflammatory mediators, since they play an important role in mediating the local response through cellular activation. The inflammatory response that occurs in the presence of an infection consists of several protective effector mechanisms that promote the microbicidal functions and in turn stimulate adaptive immunity, which contributes to reduce the damage of the tissues [38] (**Figure 1**).

IL-1β is a cytokine that is inducible through the activation of PRRs such as TLRs, by microbial products or damaged cell factors [39], once the recognition of the ligands through the receptors activates the downstream signaling pathways activating the NF-κB, activator protein (AP)-1, MAPK, and type I IFNs pathways, resulting in an upregulation of inflammatory mediators, as well as chemotactic factors [40]. IL-1β is synthesized as a precursor peptide (pro-IL-1β) that is cut to generate its mature form (mIL-1β); this process involves caspase 1, and the proenzyme (procaspase-1) requires it to be cut by the inflammasome, which is a multimeric cytosolic protein complex, composed of NLR family-pyrin domain containing 3 (NALP3) and the adapter protein containing CARD (ASC) and caspase-1; once IL-1β is cut by this complex, it binds to the IL-1R1 receptor, thus initiating the signaling that induces

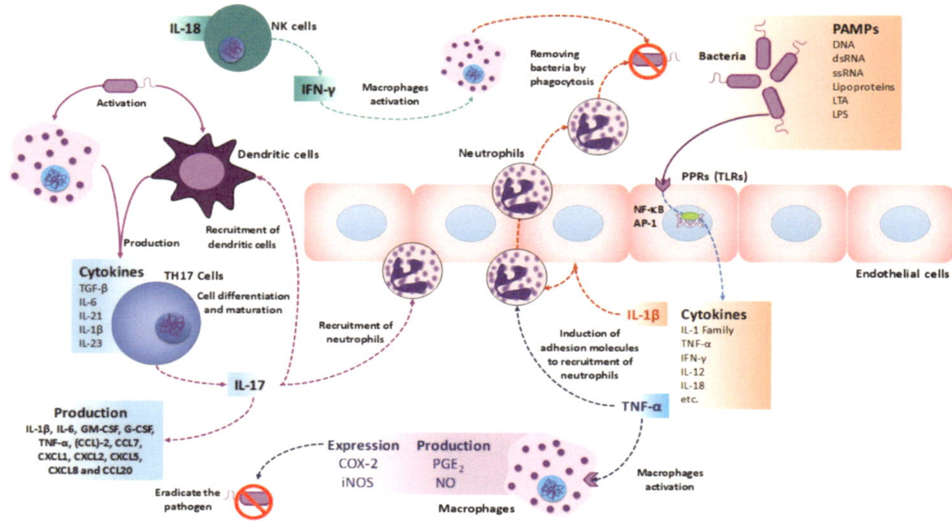

Figure 1.
Cytokines profile in bacterial infections. In response to bacterial infection, the IL-1 family cytokines, such as IL-1β, potently induces the expression of adhesion molecules in the endothelial cells and promotes the recruitment of neutrophils to the site of inflammation. TNF-α plays an important role through the recruitment of neutrophils and macrophages, besides inducing the expression of proinflammatory mediators to the site of infection. Th17 cells produce IL-17A, which induces the production of inflammatory mediators such as IL-1β, IL-6, GM-CSF, G-CSF, and TNF-α, as well as adhesion molecules. IL-18 also promotes the secretion of other proinflammatory cytokines like TNF-α, IL-1β, IL-8, and GM-CSF and consequently enhancement, migration, and activation of neutrophils during infections.

the expression of adhesion molecules in the endothelial cells and promotes the recruitment of neutrophils to the site of inflammation, as well as of the monocytes. It also has a potent stimulatory effect on phagocytosis, and it produces a chemotactic effect on leukocytes and induces the production of other inflammatory mediators of the lipid type, as well as other cytokines [41]. In vivo studies show that IL-1β is an important cytokine for the host defense against some microbial pathogens. During infection with *Staphylococcus aureus,* it was shown that the interaction of IL-1β with its receptor IL-1R plays an important role in the recruitment of neutrophils, suggesting that IL-1β is crucial for host defense against *S. aureus* and this can be transpolar to infections induced by other microorganisms [42].

Another cytokine that accompanies the IL-1β response is TNF-α, and this cytokine is produced initially during endotoxemia, as well as in response to some microbial products. TNF-α shares with IL-6 an important inflammatory property, that is, the induction of acute phase reactant protein by the liver [43]. In vivo studies show that TNF-α plays an important role in mediating clearance through the recruitment of neutrophils and macrophages to the site of infection after a bacterial intraperitoneal challenge [44], followed by an increase in the expression of COX-2, as well as inducible nitric oxide synthase (iNOS), which leads to the production of prostaglandin (PG)-E_2 and NO to eradicate the pathogen and recover homeostasis [45].

During bacterial infections, the IL-17 is another important cytokine produced. IL-17A plays an important role in the defense of the host against extracellular bacteria. The cells that are characterized mainly by producing IL-17 are a subpopulation of $CD4^+$ T cells, and their differentiation and maturation are favored by a mixture of cytokines, including transforming growth factor (TGF)-β and IL-6, IL-21 and TGF-β, or IL-1, IL-6, and IL-23 [46, 47]. The protective capacity of IL-17A against infectious agents can be mediated through several mechanisms, among these is the ability of IL-17A in the barrier surfaces to induce the production of inflammatory mediators such as IL-1β, IL-6, GM-CSF, granulocyte colony stimulating factor (G-CSF), and TNF-α, as well as adhesion molecules. IL-17A also induces the production of chemotactic factors, such as chemokine-(C-C motif)-ligand (CCL)-2, CCL7, CXCL1, CXCL2, CXCL5, and CXCL8, responsible for recruiting neutrophils and monocytes, as well as the CCL20 that is involved in the recruitment of dendritic cells, with the aim of eliminating the extracellular pathogen [48]. In vivo and in vitro studies show that signaling through TLR4 is the main mechanism by which IL-17 is induced in response to *Klebsiella pneumoniae* infection, which induces an upregulation of granulopoietic cytokines involved in the recruitment of neutrophils [49]. In mice lacking the IL-17 receptor, the recruitment of neutrophils decreased, the bacterial load increased, and survival was compromised. Whereas overexpression of IL-17 through an adenovirus, resulted in the production of cytokines mainly, macrophage inflammatory protein (MIP)-2, G-CSF, TNF-α, and IL-1β, increasing the recruitment of neutrophils, bacterial clearance and finally survival after infection with K. pneumoniae [50]. And finally, PGE2 increases the expansion of Th17 cells in an IL-1β dependent manner, thus favoring the recruitment of these cells to the site of damage. In vitro studies show that Th17 cells in the presence of PGE_2 increase the production of CCL20, thus favoring the control of infection [51].

IL-18 also promotes the secretion of other proinflammatory cytokines like TNF-α, IL-1β, IL-8, and GM-CSF and consequently enhancement, migration, and activation of neutrophils during infections. IL-18 increases the cytotoxic activity and proliferation of $CD8^+$ T and NK cells, as well as promotes the secretion of inflammatory mediators of the type TNF-α, IL-1β, IL-8, and GM-CSF, which will activate neutrophils, thus increasing their migration [38]. During a bacterial infection, IL-18 plays an important role, since it induces IFN-γ production of NK cells [52]. The IFN-γ that is produced activates macrophages and produces cytokines that induce antimicrobial pathways against intracellular and extracellular pathogens [53]. Infection with strains of lactobacillus nonpathogenic and with streptococcus pyogenes induces the expression of IL-1β, IL-6, TNF-α, IL-12, IL-18, and IFN-γ, suggesting that this type of bacterial strains induces Th1 type cytokines [54].

4. Cytokine profile in fungal infections

As well as the response to bacteria, the response against fungi also requires coordination of the innate and adaptive immune system. The innate immune system performs its effect through the cells that have the phagocytic and antigen presenting function. These cells include neutrophils, macrophages, and dendritic cells [55]. The recognition of pathogens by the immune system involves four class of PRRs: TLRs, C-type lectin receptors (CLRs), nucleotide-binding oligomerization domain-like (NOD-like) receptors (NLRs), and retinoic acid-inducible gene I (RIG-I) like receptors (RLRs) [56]. The CLRs, especially Dectin-1 and 2, play an important role in the pathogen recognition from *Candida spp.*; this is because the cell wall is made up of mannoproteins with O-glycosylated oligosaccharide and N-glycosylated polysaccharide moieties, with an inner layer of chitin and β (1, 3) and β (1, 6) glucans are recognized and initiate a downstream signaling through these receptors, which leads to activation of the transcription factor NF-κB and other signaling pathways that induce the production of pro-inflammatory cytokines such as IL-6, IL-1β, and IL-23 that induce the Th17 cytokines [57] (**Figure 2**).

The recognition of fungi by phagocytic cells occurs mainly through the detection of cell wall components such as mannan, β-glucan, phosphocholine, β-1,6 glucan, and even internal components such as DNA can be recognized [58, 59]. The recruitment and activation of phagocytic cells are mediated through the induction

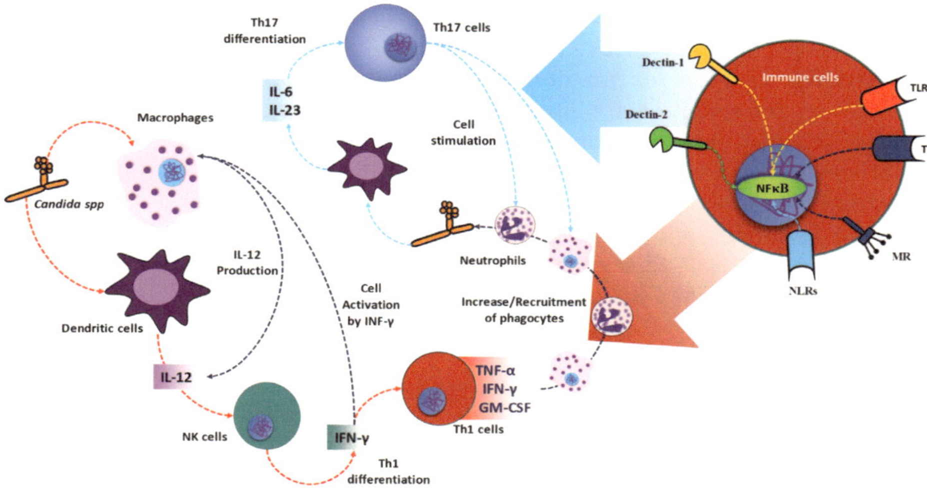

Figure 2.
Cytokines profile in fungal infections. The PRRs recognize fungal PAMPs and initiate a downstream signaling, which leads to the activation of the NF-κB and other signaling pathways inducing the production of cytokines such as IL-6, IL-1β, IL-12, TNF-α, GM-CSF, IFN-γ, and IL-23. These cytokines induce the differentiation of Th1 and Th17 immune responses against fungi infection, stimulating the migration, adherence, and phagocytosis of neutrophils and macrophages.

of proinflammatory cytokines, chemokines, and complement components. Fungi are killed by oxidative and nonoxidative mechanisms and antimicrobial peptides. These activities are influenced by the action of cytokines such as IFN-γ [59]. This cytokine produced mainly by T and NK cells stimulates the migration, adherence, and phagocytosis of neutrophils and macrophages and production of opsonizing antibodies and maintains a Th1 response as a protective response against fungi. It also induces a classical activation of macrophages that is important to stop the growth of intracellular fungal pathogens [60]. The Th1 response occurs through the release of proinflammatory cytokines IFN-γ, TNF-α, and GM-CSF, increasing the permeability in the tissue, as well as the phagocytic cells at the site of infection to efficiently clean the infection [61] (**Figure 2**).

Another important cytokine in immunity against fungi is IL-12, and this cytokine is considered the main cytokine that induces IFN-γ production. IL-12 is produced by monocytes, macrophages, and dendritic cells, in response to microbial products, and acts on NK and T cells to induce IFN-γ. On the other hand, the late secretion of IL-12 in the lymph nodes induces naive T cells to produce IFN-γ and therefore amounting a Th1 response is promoted [62]. The ability of IFN-γ to increase the production of IL-12 forms a positive feedback during the inflammatory process and the Th1 response, and this interferon in turn activates monocytes and macrophages to induce the production of IL-12 [63] (**Figure 2**). Studies in $Il12p35^{-/-}$ and $IFN\text{-}\gamma^{-/-}$ mice show an increase in susceptibility to infections with *Candida albicans*, and this suggests that IL-12 and the Th1 responses play an important role in controlling *Candida* infection [64]. On the other hand, neutrophils kill the extracellular and intracellular fungi through effector mechanism that includes the production of reactive oxygen and nitrogen species, as well as the release of hydrolytic enzymes and their granules containing antimicrobial peptides [65].

IL-23 is a member of the IL-12 family and plays a central role in the expansion of Th17 cells as well as their function, composed of a p19 and p40 subunit that shares it with IL-12 [66, 67]. IL-23 is produced primarily by dendritic cells, the binding of β-glucan to Dectin-1 activates the syk-CARD-9 signaling pathway leading to the production of IL-23, which promotes the Th17 response, through the differentiation of naïve CD4+ T cells into Th17 cells and the release of IL-17A, IL-17F and IL-22 in response to infections caused by mucosal fungi [68]. These cytokines in conjunction with IL-23 have various functions in the body from a proinflammatory, anti-inflammatory, or regulatory activity, which depends on the type of microorganism, the site of infection, and the immunological status of the host (**Figure 2**). In vivo studies have shown that mice deficient of the IL-17 receptor (IL-17RA$^{-/-}$) cannot limit systemic candidiasis, as well as oropharyngeal candidiasis, being more susceptible to developing mucocutaneous candidiasis, suggesting that the Th17 lineage strongly acts through IL-17, regulating the expansion, recruitment, and migration of neutrophils, as well as CXC-chemokines and antimicrobial proteins such as β-defensin 3 [66, 69].

5. Cytokine profile in viral infections

In viral infections, the cytokines are implicated to establish an antiviral state as the unspecific first line of defense and virus-specific response. This process initiates through recognition of viral molecules by PRRs, which can be found as transmembrane receptors or in different intracellular compartment. The receptor undergoes a structural change, activating a route of signalization in the cytoplasm that end with the activation of cytoplasmic transcription factors that translocate into the nuclei to promote the expression of different cytokines. Depending of the virus and the type of cell, the type of cytokine produced may vary [70, 71].

5.1 Pattern recognition receptors versus virus

Viruses can infect virtually all cells of an organism. Epithelial, endothelial, fibroblasts, neurons, as well as innate and adaptive immune cells can be infected. PRRs are present in both nonhematopoietic origin cell and immune cells. Some PRRs recognize viral proteins, but other can detect viral single or double RNA or DNA. In human, there are 10 TLRs distributed in plasmatic membrane and endosome membranes. Of them, TLR-2 and TLR-4 can detect viral surface glycoprotein before the viral penetration. Others like TLR-3, TLR-8, and TLR-9 sense different types of viral nucleic acids in endosomes during virus entering. TLR-8 senses genomic ssRNA, TLR-3 senses dsRNA, and TLR-9 detects nonmethylated CpG viral DNA [72, 73]. Another type of receptors that sense viral RNA are the RNA helicases receptors like RIG-I and melanoma differentiation-associated gene 5 (MDA5) [71, 74]. These receptors have been demonstrated to detect viral dsRNA. This dsRNA can be genomic or an intermediate form during replication, which is formed, virtually, for all virus of single or double RNA during viral replication. However, there is evidence that some dsRNA replicative intermediators can translocate to endosomes where TLR can sense and trigger the signalization way [75].

5.2 Cytokines produced in viral infections

There are many cytokines with distinct functions. All of them are molecules with less than 20 KDa and can be pleiotropic or redundant, and also, they can synergize or antagonize each other. However, all of them are produced to ensure the virus elimination through the regulation of the immune response against the virus [76]. The process includes detection of the pathogen, signal to neighbor cells, activation and differentiation of innate immune cells, production of adhesion molecules on endothelial cell for extravasation of immune circulating cell, chemotactic molecules to attract cell to the infection foci, increase of phagocytosis, and activation of adaptive cells to specifically eliminate infected cells and extracellular virus [77].

Cytokine network against viruses starts with some cytokines produced by virus-infected cells (**Figure 3**). Epithelial cell can produce IFN, IL-8, IL-6, IL-1, GM-CSF [78, 79], TNFα [80], IL-18 [81], IL-12 [82], IL-2 [83], and IL-23 [84, 85]. The role of these cytokines is varied, IFN induces an antiviral state, and IL-8 is a potent inflammatory attracting phagocyte cell to the site of infection. IL-1 can promote apoptosis, and it is proinflammatory and chemotactic to neutrophils. GM-CSF is a hematopoietic grow factor that recruits various immune cells to host defense [76, 86]. Moreover, in the infection course, varies cytokines are also produced by innate and adaptive cell that can also be infected or activated. In filovirus infection, IL-1β, IL-5, IL-8, and IL-18, as well as varies chemokines like MIP-1α and β, monocyte chemoattractant protein 1 (MCP-1), and IFN-γ–inducible protein 10 (IP10) among others are produced [77]. In influenza virus infection, TNF-α, IL-1 α and β, and IL-6 and IL-8 are produced [87], and hepatitis C virus can promote the expression of IL-6, IL-8, MIP-1α, and MIP-1β and IL-1 [88], while rotavirus can induce the production of IFN, IL-8, IL-6, IL-1 [89], TNF-α [80], IL-18 [81], IL-12 [82], IL-2 [83], and IL-23 [84, 85]. Thus, the infected cell can upregulate multiple cytokine genes involved in different process as activation of NK, macrophages, and dendritic cells. Increasing the production of cytokines that serve as bridge between innate and adaptive response. In the inflammation process, virus-infected cells produce and secrete proinflammatory cytokines like IL-1, IL-6, IL-8, TNF [70] and

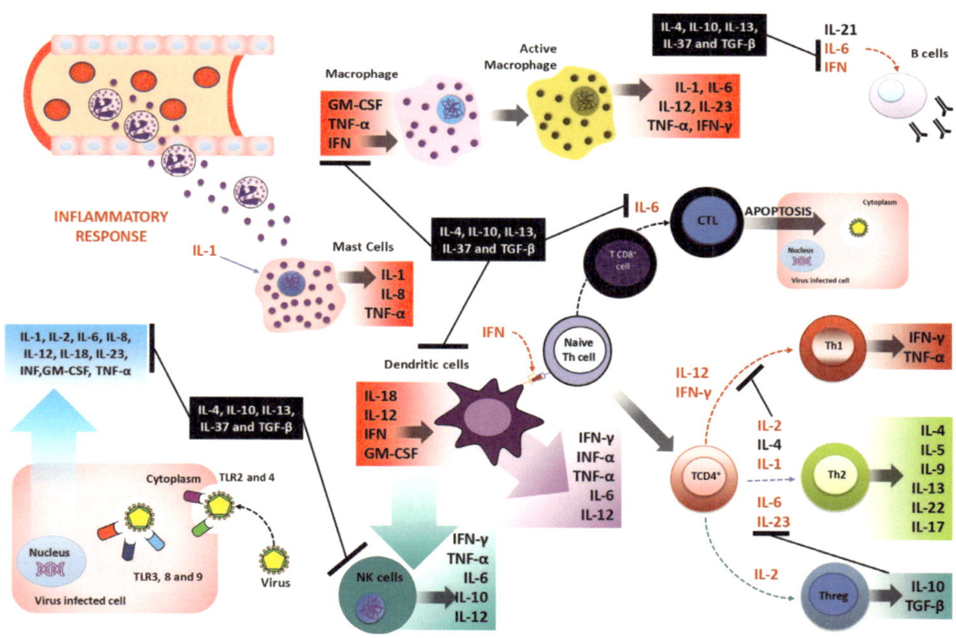

Figure 3.
Cytokines profile in viral infections. The immune response against viruses initiates through recognition of viral molecules by PRRs. These PRRs can activate a signal system culminating in the activation of transcription factors involved in the establishment of an antiviral state and an inflammation process. Cytokine network against viruses start with some cytokines produced by virus infected cells, such as IFNs, IL-8, IL-6, IL-1, GM-CSF, TNFα, IL-18, IL-12, IL-2 and IL-23, inducing a potent inflammatory response, attracting and activating phagocyte cells (e.g. neutrophils, macrophages, dendritic cells), mast cells and NK cells, to the site of infection. Furthermore, these cytokines are involved in the induction of an immune response type Th1/TCL with the purpose of eliminate infected cells and extracellular virus while cytokines such as IL-4, IL-10, IL-13, IL-37, and TGF-β modulate the immune response to a Th2 and Th17 phenotype, which produce immunomodulatory and anti-inflammatory actions.

IFN. These cytokines can be involved in the early defense of the organism. They can activate cells present in the site of infection, and they can recruit leukocyte cells from circulating system through inflammation process (**Figure 3**).

5.3 Cytokines' role in viral infection

IFN is a pleiotropic cytokine produced by virus infection. Although there are three types of IFN called type I (α/β), type II (γ) and type III (λ). Type I IFN plays an important role in control early viral infections. The role of type I IFN is to interfere with viral replication through activating the expression of antiviral molecules. Once IFN is secreted, it can act in autocrine or paracrine (like other cytokines) way, interacting with interferon receptor to induce the production of an antiviral state in the infected and noninfected neighboring cells, inhibiting different step of viral replication [76]. Also, IFN promotes the production of cytokines like IL-12, IL-6, IFN-γ, and TNF-α in innate cells including NK cells and macrophages [90]. Another function of IFN is to enhance differentiation of dendritic cells [91] and promote the antigen presentation [90] to stimulate T and B cells [92], which is redundant with the function of the IL-12 and IL-18 [93, 94]. NK cells are activated by synergism between type 1 IFNs and IL-12. However, cytokines such as IL-10, IL-6, IL-4, IL-13, and TGF-β suppress the actions of IFN, and these cytokines are known for their immunomodulatory and anti-inflammatory actions [95].

TNF-α is other pleiotropic cytokine produced by also nonhematopoietic infected cells and innate and adaptive immune cells, including macrophages, dendritic cells, natural killer, and T and B lymphocytes after being activated [96]. This cytokine can activate the production of adhesion molecules in endothelial cells and promote the extravasation of neutrophils, monocytes, and others immune cells to be attracted to infection foci. TNF also can participate in apoptosis through activating caspases. TNF-α, together with IFN-γ, acts on macrophages, inducing the production of superoxide anions and oxygen and nitrogen radicals [97]. Macrophages can also produce cytokines such as IL-1, IL-6, IL-23, IL-12, and more TNF-α [95].

IL-1 was the first interleukin to be identified and is a pleiotropic cytokine, and it acts synergically with IL-6 on the central nervous system, inducing fever by activation of the hypothalamus-pituitary-adrenal (HPA) axis [98]. This molecule also activates mast cells and induces histamine production, acting as a vasodilator, thus increases the permeability of the membrane [99]. Also, IL-1 is chemotactic factor that induces the passage of neutrophils to the site of infection. This chemotactic function is redundant with the action of IL-8, also known as chemokine CXCL8 [86] also produced by the infected cell. There are cytokines that antagonize these functions of IL-1 such as IL-10, IL-4, and IL-13 recognized for their anti-inflammatory actions [100].

Another pleiotropic cytokine is IL-18, first described as "interferon-γ-inducing factor" and member of IL-1 family. This interleukin and type I IFN are recognized by dendritic cells and trigger a signaling pathway through TRF6 and induce the expression of $CD11b^+$ in the surface of the cell [94]. These activated cells can express cytokines like IL-12, IL-6, IFN-γ, TNFα, and IFN-α, which also participates in other hematopoietic cells [101, 102]. IL-18 also participates synergistically with interleukin 12 on the activation of NK cells [93], stimulating the expression of CD25 and CD69 molecules, promoting their proliferation and cytotoxic capacity, respectively. Once activated, NK cells can induce apoptosis in virus-infected cells and produce other cytokines such as IL-12, IL-6, IL-10, IFN-γ, and TNF-α. Within the cytokines that block these functions of IL-18 are IL-37, IL-10, and TGF-β [103].

IL-6 is a soluble mediator with a pleiotropic effect on inflammation, immune response, and hematopoiesis. IL-6 is an important mediator of fever and of the acute phase response, which is redundant with IL-1 and TFN-α and promotes the differentiation of cytotoxic T lymphocytes, which induce the death of infected cells by osmotic lysis [104]. IL-6 synergistically with IL-23 participates in the differentiation of Th17 [105], through the production of RORγt. Once activated, Th17 induces inflammatory response through the expression of cytokines as IL-17 and IL-22. IL-6 also promotes the proliferation of B cells by binding to a complex of receptors (gp80, CD126, and CD130) [106] and, like IL-21 [107], induces the differentiation of plasma cells stimulating the antibody production [108]. However, there exist antagonist cytokines like IL-10, IL-13, and TGF-β that inhibit all these functions of the IL-6 [103].

IL-12, also known as a T cell-stimulating factor, which together with IFN-γ, promotes differentiation of Th1 cells by activation of T-bet, and these cells can activate macrophages through expression of other cytokines like IFN and TNF, amplifying the produced immune response [109]. Although, there is evidence that viruses may selectively induce IFN production and Th1 differentiation even in the absence of IL-12 [110].

IL-2 participates in the differentiation and proliferation of Th2 (redundant with IL-4) and Treg cells by the expression of GATA-3 and FOXP3, respectively [111, 112]. Th2 cells can express IL-4, IL-5, IL-9, and IL-13, which also have pleiotropic effects in promoting type 2 effector mechanisms, such as B cells secretion of immunoglobulins, eosinophilia, mastocytosis, and M2 macrophage polarization [113]. T_{reg} cells regulate the immune response, suppressing T-cell activation [114]. T_{reg} and Th2 are known for their immunomodulatory and anti-inflammatory actions [95]. Finally, GM-CSF stimulates the generation of dendritic cells and participates in polarization of macrophages M1 [115]. Moreover, GM-CSF has also been associated with Th2 immunity and therefore M2 polarization. GM-CSF is considered a pleiotropic cytokine with inflammatory and anti-inflammatory functions [116].

6. Cytokine profile in parasitic infections

In parasitic infections is difficult to generalize about the mechanisms of anti-parasitic immunity because there is a great variety of different parasites that have different morphology and reside in different locations of tissues and hosts during their life cycles [117]. In this section of the chapter, we will talk about the immune response against protozoa and helminths, two of the main parasites of medical importance for human health.

6.1 Immune system activation by parasitic protozoan infections

Protozoan parasites are much larger and more complex pathogens than viruses or bacteria and have developed additional and sophisticated strategies to escape the immune attack of the host. Currently, 30% of humans suffer parasitic protozoan infections worldwide. Life cycles of protozoans generally involve several stages of specific antigenicity, which facilitates their survival and propagation within different cells, tissues, and hosts. Frequently, the host fails to eliminate protozoan infections, which often results in a chronic disease or inapparent infections, in which the host continues to act as a reservoir of parasites [118].

The immune defense mechanisms against protozoan parasites frequently involve several immune cells such as neutrophils, macrophages, and NK cells that mediate the innate response against extracellular protozoan parasites. NK cell and cytokine-activated macrophages are central to the innate response to intracellular parasites. Innate cytokine and dendritic cell responses also play a critical role in the induction of adaptive immunity [119].

During the initial stage of parasitic protozoan infections, intestinal epithelial cells (IECs) bind and recognize PAMPs through PRRs [120] such as TLR-2 and TLR-4 [121], which activates NF-κB and leads to the production of proinflammatory cytokines [122], including IL-1β, IL-6, IL-8, IL-12, IFN-γ, and TNF-α [123, 124], which induces the activation of a Th1 type response [125]. IFN-γ is involved in clearance of infection, through the activation of neutrophils and macrophages (**Figure 4**) [126–132]. It has been also shown that IFN-γ-producing $CD4^+$ T cells are involved protection in vaccinated mice [133]. Several studies suggest a role for IFN-γ in the pathogenesis of parasitic protozoan infections. In both humans and animal models, the production of high levels of IFN-γ is associated with resistance to infection [134–136], while low levels of IFN-γ are associated with an increased susceptibility to infection. Therefore, it is considered highly probable that IFN-γ provides protection against infection by activation of neutrophils and/or macrophages [125]. The production of reactive oxygen species (ROS) and NO through the complex of NADPH oxidase and iNOS, respectively, plays a critical role in the elimination of protozoan parasites [131, 132]. In experimental studies, infection protection was mediated by IFN-γ from NK T cells (NKT), while TNF-α is produced by increased tissue damage [137, 138], together with IL-1 and IL-8 [139] (**Figure 4**).

On the other hand, the antigenic exposure of protozoan parasites activates a Th2-type immune response by the host, inducing the production of anti-inflammatory cytokines such as IL-4, IL-10 [125], IL-5 and IL-13, which try to attenuate the Th1 type response characterized also by the INF-γ production, leading to upregulation of Th2 cytokine responses (IL-4, IL-5, and IL-13) and Th17 (IL-17), suppressing the production of Th1 cytokines [140] (**Figure 4**). In addition, another cytokine of anti-inflammatory importance is TGF-β, which acts in a synergistic manner to counteract this Th1 type response, activating macrophages which produce

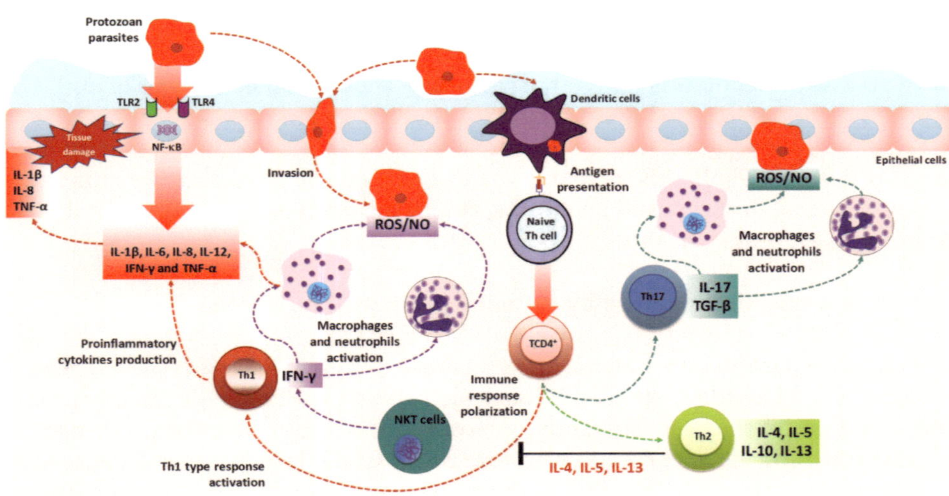

Figure 4.
Cytokines profile in parasitic protozoan infections. The immune defense mechanisms against protozoan parasites involve several immune cells such as neutrophils, macrophages, NK cells, and $CD4^+$ T cells. These cells are capable to produce proinflammatory cytokines, such as IL-1β, IL-6, IL-8, IL-12, IFN-γ, and TNF-α, promoting type 1 immune response. Likewise, protozoan parasites activate a Th2-type immune response, producing anti-inflammatory cytokines such as IL-4, IL-10, IL-5, and IL-13, suppressing the production of Th1 cytokines.

NO, through iNOS, for the elimination of the parasite [138]. Therefore, Th1-type cytokine response is characterized mainly by the production of IFN-γ, whereas susceptibility to tissue damage by protozoan parasites is critically dependent on a Th2-type cytokine response mediated mainly by IL-4.

6.2 Immune system activation by parasitic helminth infection

More than two billion people around the world are infected with helminth parasites. Parasitic helminth infections are a major public health problem worldwide due to their ability to cause great morbidity and socioeconomic loss [141, 142].

The immune response against helminth parasites is characterized by the induction of an early Th1-type immune response, with the subsequent predominance of a Th2 type immune response, resulting in a mixture of both Th1/Th2 immune responses [143, 144], which depend on the CD4$^+$ T cells [145]. The CD4$^+$ T cells have a key role in the establishment of the cytokine environment during helminth parasite infection, thus directing their differentiation either by suppressing or favoring the inflammatory response at the intestinal level, which is crucial for the elimination of the parasite [146] (**Figure 5**).

PAMPs derived from helminth parasites induce the activation and maturation of dendritic cells [147, 148], promoting the development of the Th1 immune response [149], which results in a significant increase of Th1 cytokines such as IL-12 [150–152], INF-γ [149–153], IL-1β [152, 154], and TNF-α [150–152, 155] (**Figure 5**). However, in recent years, several studies have shown that this immune response of Th1 type favors infection by helminth parasites. On the one hand, IL-12 and INF-γ are two important cytokines against infection by helminth parasites, since they participate in the polarization of the Th1 type immune response [149–151, 153]. However, exogenous IL-12 is capable of suppressing intestinal mastocytosis, delaying the parasite expulsion, and increasing the parasite burden at the muscular level [156]. INF-γ induces the expression of iNOS, activates transcription factors such as NF-κB [157], and regulates the production of pro-inflammatory cytokines such as TNF-α [158]. Studies have shown that TNF-α is a cytokine that is produced during

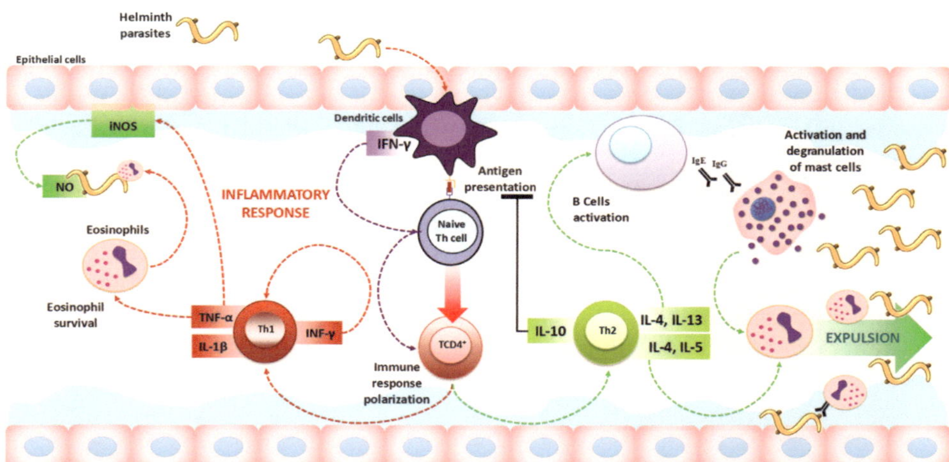

Figure 5.
Cytokines profile in parasitic helminth infection. The immune response against helminth parasites is characterized by the induction of an early Th1 type immune response, which results in a significant increase of Th1 cytokines such as IL-12, INF-γ, IL-1β, and TNF-α. Then, there is a subsequent predominance of a Th2 type immune response characterized by the release of IL-4, IL-5, IL-10, and IL-13 favoring helminth parasites expulsion.

intestinal infection by helminth parasites [150, 151, 159], which is necessary in the protection against the parasite through the Th2 immune response [160]. However, several studies have associated the production of TNF-α with the development of intestinal pathology during infection by helminth parasites [155, 161, 162]. One of the effects of TNF-α is the iNOS expression and consequently the NO production [163–165]. Helminth parasite antigens are capable to induce the expression of iNOS, with the subsequent production of NO [166], which acts mainly as an effector molecule against both extracellular and intracellular parasites [167]. Studies in iNOS knockout mice infected with helminth parasites, showed a reduction in the expression of Th2 cytokines (IL-4, IL-5), a reduced humoral response (IgG and IgE), with a decrease in mastocytosis. However, no significant difference was observed in the helminth parasite expulsion, although iNOS knockout mice showed a decrease in intestinal pathology compared to wild-type animals. These results suggest that NO is not required for the helminth parasite expulsion, but its production is responsible for the intestinal pathology [155, 168]. With respect to IL-1β, it is well known that it participates in the intestinal inflammatory response in the helminth parasites infection, observing high levels during intestinal infection. However, until now, the role of IL-1β is not well understood [159].

With respect to the Th2 type immune response, in vitro studies have shown that helminth parasite antigens are capable of dendritic cells activating, inducing the synthesis of Th2 cytokines such as IL-4, IL-5, IL-10, and IL-13 [147, 149, 153, 169]. Likewise, studies in in vivo models have shown that helminth parasites infection is a significant increase in the synthesis of IL-4, IL-5, IL-10, and IL-13 [150, 151, 159, 170] (**Figure 5**). IL-10 may suppress antigen presentation by dendritic cells and inhibition of IL-12 secretion. In addition, helminth parasite antigens increased both IL-4 and IL-10 production derived from Th2 cells with a decrease in INF-γ production, polarizing the immune response to a strong Th2 cellular immune response, protective and responsible for the helminth parasite expulsion [143]. IL-10 is a Th2 cytokine, which is necessary for a successful intestinal immune response. This is because the absence or decrease of IL-10 causes a significant delay in the helminth parasite expulsion and an increase in the parasite burden [171]. IL-4 and IL-13 induce muscle cells hypercontractility of the jejunum and intestinal mastocytosis, promoting the helminth parasite expulsion [161, 172]. In IL-4/IL-13 mice deficient, a reduction in the helminth parasite expulsion, mastocytosis, and development of intestinal pathology was observed [161, 162, 173, 174]. Therefore, these studies suggest that IL-4 and IL-13 can regulate the induction of the protective Th2 immune response and intestinal inflammation, both associated with the helminth parasite expulsion [162]. During the Th2 immune response, the cytokines such as IL-4, IL-5, and IL-13 stimulate IgE synthesis [175], inducing mast cell and eosinophil hyperplasia [176], triggering immediate hypersensitivity reactions, and promoting the helminth parasite expulsion from the intestine [177]. However, mast cells and eosinophils are involved in tissue damage, thus promoting the inflammatory response. It suggests that the protective role of the Th2 type immune response is not sufficient facing the challenge against helminth parasite infections, as it contributes to the development of immunopathology [178] (**Figure 5**).

7. Conclusion

Although cytokines are produced with the purpose of modulating the immune response against infections caused by microorganisms, such as bacteria, fungi, viruses, and parasites, there is evidence that these microorganisms can induce cytokine production with bad prognostic to host recovery. In this sense, overproduction of inflammatory cytokines may be responsible for the severe damage observed in many microorganism infections. For this reason, a better understanding over the cytokine balance related to diseases by microorganisms is required to avoid severe damage against the organism caused by overreaction of the immune system.

Acknowledgements

We thank the authors who collaborated in the writing of this chapter: Dr. José Luis Muñoz, Dr. Juan Francisco Contreras, Dr. Oscar Gutiérrez, Dra. Paola Trinidad Villalobos, Dra. Viridiana Elizabeth Hernández and Luis Guillermo; as well as the Universities involved: Cuauhtémoc University Aguascalientes, Autonomous University of Nuevo Leon, and University of Guadalajara. We also thank the financial support for chapter publication.

Conflict of interest

We have no conflict of interest related to this work.

Author details

José Luis Muñoz-Carrillo[1*], Juan Francisco Contreras-Cordero[2], Oscar Gutiérrez-Coronado[3], Paola Trinidad Villalobos-Gutiérrez[3], Luis Guillermo Ramos-Gracia[4] and Viridiana Elizabeth Hernández-Reyes[1]

1 Faculty of Odontology, School of Biomedical Sciences of the Cuauhtémoc University Aguascalientes, Aguascalientes, Mexico

2 Laboratory of Immunology and Virology, Faculty of Biological Sciences of the Autonomous University of Nuevo Leon, San Nicolás de Los Garza, Nuevo León, Mexico

3 Laboratory of Immunology, Department of Earth and Life Sciences, University Center of Lagos de Moreno of the University of Guadalajara, Lagos de Moreno, Jalisco, Mexico

4 Faculty of Medicine, School of Biomedical Sciences of the Cuauhtémoc University Aguascalientes, Aguascalientes, Mexico

*Address all correspondence to: mcbjlmc@gmail.com

References

[1] Silva-Barrios S, Stäger S. Protozoan parasites and type I IFNs. Frontiers in Immunology. 2017;**8**:14. DOI: 10.3389/fimmu.2017.00014

[2] Grignani G, Maiolo A. Cytokines and hemostasis. Haematologica. 2000;**85**(9):967-972

[3] Carson WF, Kunkel SL. Type I and II cytokine superfamilies in inflammatory responses. In: Cavaillon JM, Singer M, editors. Inflammation: From Molecular and Cellular Mechanisms to the Clinic. Weinheim, Germany: Wiley-VCH Verlag GmbH & Co. KGaA; 2017. pp. 587-618. DOI: 10.1002/9783527692156.ch24

[4] O'Shea JJ, Gadina M, Siegel RM. Cytokines and cytokine receptors. In: Rich RR, Fleisher TA, Shearer WT, Schroeder HW, Frew AJ, Weyand CM, editors. Clinical Immunology. 5th ed. London: Content Repository Only; 2019. pp. 127-155.e1. DOI: 10.1016/B978-0-7020-6896-6.00009-0

[5] Muñoz Carrillo JL, Castro García FP, Gutiérrez Coronado O, Moreno García MA, Contreras Cordero JF. Physiology and pathology of innate immune response against pathogens. In: Rezaei N, editor. Physiology and Pathology of Immunology. London: InTech; 2017. pp. 99-134. DOI: 10.5772/intechopen.70556

[6] Dinarello CA. Biologic basis for interleukin-1 in disease. Blood. 1996;**87**(6):2095-2147

[7] Dinarello CA. Immunological and inflammatory functions of the interleukin-1 family. Annual Review of Immunology. 2009;**27**:519-550. DOI: 10.1146/annurev.immunol.021908.132612

[8] Sims JE, Smith DE. The IL-1 family: Regulators of immunity. Nature Reviews. Immunology. 2010;**10**(2):89-102. DOI: 10.1038/nri2691

[9] Boraschi D, Tagliabue A. The interleukin-1 receptor family. Seminars in Immunology. 2013;**25**(6):394-407. DOI: 10.1016/j.smim.2013.10.023

[10] Dinarello C. IL-1 superfamily and inflammasome. In: Cavaillon JM, Singer M, editors. Inflammation: From Molecular and Cellular Mechanisms to the Clinic. Weinheim, Germany: Wiley-VCH Verlag GmbH & Co. KGaA; 2017. pp. 477-528. DOI: 10.1002/9783527692156.ch20

[11] Gay NJ, Keith FJ. Drosophila Toll and IL-1 receptor. Nature. 1991;**351**(6325):355-356. DOI: 10.1038/351355b0

[12] Pappu BP, Borodovsky A, Zheng TS, Yang X, Wu P, Dong X, et al. TL1A–DR3 interaction regulates Th17 cell function and Th17-mediated autoimmune disease. The Journal of Experimental Medicine. 2008;**205**(5):1049-1062. DOI: 10.1084/jem.20071364

[13] Garlanda C, Riva F, Bonavita E, Mantovani A. Negative regulatory receptors of the IL-1 family. Seminars in Immunology. 2013;**25**(6):408-415. DOI: 10.1016/j.smim.2013.10.019

[14] Aggarwal BB, Gupta SC, Kim JH. Historical perspectives on tumor necrosis factor and its superfamily: 25 years later, a golden journey. Blood. 2012;**119**(3):651-665. DOI: 10.1182/blood-2011-04-325225

[15] Cuzzocrea S. TNF Superfamily. In: Cavaillon JM, Singer M, editors. Inflammation: From Molecular and Cellular Mechanisms to the Clinic. Weinheim, Germany: Wiley-VCH Verlag GmbH & Co. KGaA; 2017. pp. 529-547. DOI: 10.1002/9783527692156.ch21

[16] Croft M. The role of TNF superfamily members in T-cell function and diseases. Nature Reviews.

Immunology. 2009;**9**(4):271-285. DOI: 10.1038/nri2526

[17] Carswell EA, Old LJ, Kassel RL, Green S, Fiore N, Williamson B. An endotoxin-induced serum factor that causes necrosis of tumors. Proceedings of the National Academy of Sciences of the United States of America. 1975;**72**(9):3666-3670

[18] Yao Z, Fanslow WC, Seldin MF, Rousseau AM, Painter SL, Comeau MR, et al. Herpesvirus saimiri encodes a new cytokine, IL-17, which binds to a novel cytokine receptor. Journal of Immunology. 2011;**187**(9):4392-4402

[19] Korn T, Bettelli E, Oukka M, Kuchroo VK. IL-17 and Th17 cells. Annual Review of Immunology. 2009;**27**:485-517. DOI: 10.1146/annurev.immunol.021908.132710

[20] Monteleone G, Marafini I. Troncone E interleukin-17 A-E. In: Cavaillon JM, Singer M, editors. Inflammation: From Molecular and Cellular Mechanisms to the Clinic. Weinheim, Germany: Wiley-VCH Verlag GmbH & Co. KGaA; 2017. pp. 549-572. DOI: 10.1002/9783527692156.ch22

[21] Tanaka T, Narazaki M, Kishimoto T. IL-6 Superfamily. In: Cavaillon JM, Singer M, editors. Inflammation: From Molecular and Cellular Mechanisms to the Clinic. Weinheim, Germany: Wiley-VCH Verlag GmbH & Co. KGaA; 2017. pp. 573-589. DOI: 10.1002/9783527692156.ch23

[22] Hibi M, Nakajima K, Hirano T. IL-6 cytokine family and signal transduction: A model of the cytokine system. Journal of Molecular Medicine. 1996;**74**:1-12. DOI: 10.1007/BF0020 2068

[23] Hirano T, Ishihara K, Hibi M. Roles of STAT3 in mediating the cell growth, differentiation and survival signals relayed through the IL-6 family of cytokine receptors. Oncogene. 2009;**19**(21):2548-2556. DOI: 10.1038/sj.ocn.1203551

[24] Rose-John S. Interleukin-6 family cytokines. Cold Spring Harbor Perspectives in Biology. 2018;**10**(2):1-17. DOI: 10.1101/cshperspect.a028415

[25] Tanaka T, Narazaki M, Kishimoto T. Therapeutic targeting of the interleukin-6 receptor. Annual Review of Pharmacology and Toxicology. 2012;**52**:199-219. DOI: 10.1146/annurev-pharmtox-010611-134715

[26] Tanaka T, Narazaki M, Kishimoto T. IL-6 in inflammation, immunity, and disease. Cold Spring Harbor Perspectives in Biology. 2014;**6**(10):1-16. DOI: 10.1101/cshperspect.a016295

[27] Owen J, Punt J, Stranford S, Jones P. Kuby Inmmunology. 7th ed. México: Editorial McGrawHill; 2014. pp. 116-123. ISBN: 978-607-15-1126-3

[28] Smith KA. The structure of IL2 bound to the three chains of the IL2 receptor and how signaling occurs. Medical Immunology. 2006;**5**:3. DOI: 10.1186/1476-9433-5-3

[29] Sinobiological. Cytokine Families [Internet]. 2017. Available form: https://www.sinobiological.com/Cytokine-Families-Cytokine-Family-a-5797.html [Accessed: May 29, 2018]

[30] Sinobiological. Interleukin 2 & Receptor [Internet]. 2017. Available form: https://www.sinobiological.com/IL-2-Interleukin-2-Receptor-a-6073.html [Accessed: May 31, 2018]

[31] Thermo Fisher Scientific. Interferon (IFN) Cell Signaling Pathway [Internet]. 2017. Available from: https://www.thermofisher.com/mx/es/home/life-science/cell-analysis/signaling-pathways/interferon/interferon-overview.html [Accessed: Jun 1, 2018]

[32] Wolff K, Goldsmith L, Katz S, Gilchrest B, Paller A, Leffell D. Fitzpatrick Dermatologia en Medicina General. 7th ed. México: Editorial Editorial Medica Panamericana; 2009. pp. 124-125. ISBN: 978-950-06-1703-1

[33] González M, Ordónez A. La Astenia Tumoral. 1st ed. Editorial Medica Panamericana. México, 2004. pp. 32-35. ISBN: 84-7903-962-0

[34] Michael FT. Innate immune responses to infection. The Journal of Allergy and Clinical Immunology. 2005;**116**(2):241-249. DOI: 10.1016/j.jaci.2005.05.036

[35] Dejan B, Vuk RV, Suzana P, Predrag D, Milan Z, Ivana N, et al. Cytokine profile in chronic hepatitis C: An observation. Cytokine. 2017;**96**:185-188. DOI: 10.1016/j.cyto.2017.04.008

[36] Andrea JW, David MU. Peptidoglycan recognition by the innate immune system. Nature Reviews. Immunology. 2018;**8**(4):243-254. DOI: 10.1038/nri.2017.136

[37] Kawai T, Akira S. The roles of TLRs, RLRs and NLRs in pathogen recognition. International Immunology. 2009;**21**(4):317-337. DOI: 10.1093/intimm/dxp017

[38] Manoranjan S, Ivonne CO, Laura B, Fabio R. Role of the inflammasome, IL-1*β* and IL-18 in bacterial infections. The Scientific World Journal. 2011;**11**:2037-2050. DOI: 10.1100/2011/212680

[39] Borthwick LA. The IL-1 cytokine family and its role in inflammation and fibrosis in the lung. Seminars in Immunopathology. 2016;**38**(4):517-534. DOI: 10.1007/s00281-016-0559-z

[40] Broggi A, Granucci F. Microbe- and danger-induced inflammation. Molecular Immunology. 2015;**63**(2):127-133. DOI: 10.1016/j.molimm.2014.06.037

[41] Biondo C, Mancuso G, Midiri A, Signorino G, Domina M, Lanza Cariccio V, et al. Essential role of interleukin-1 signaling in host defenses against group B streptococcus. MBio. 2014;**5**(5):e01428-e014214. DOI: 10.1128/mBio.01428-14

[42] Miller LS, Pietras EM, Uricchio LH, Hirano K, Rao S, Lin H, et al. Inflammasome-mediated production of IL-1β is required for neutrophil recruitment against *Staphylococcus aureus* in vivo. Journal of Immunology. 2007;**179**(10):6933-6942. DOI: 10.4049/jimmunol.179.10.6933

[43] Arango DG, Descoteaux A. Macrophage cytokines: Involvement in immunity and infectious diseases. Frontiers in Immunology. 2014;**5**:491-502. DOI: 10.3389/fimmu.2014.00491

[44] Malaviya R, Abraham SN. Role of mast cell leukotrienes in neutrophil recruitment and bacterial clearance in infectious peritonitis. Journal of Leukocyte Biology. 2000;**67**(6):841-846. DOI: 10.1002/jlb.67.6.841

[45] Dinarello CA. Proinflammatory cytokines. Chest. 2000;**118**(2):503-508. DOI: 10.1378/chest.118.2.503

[46] Harrington LE, Hatton RD, Mangan PR, Turner H, Murphy TL, Murphy KM, et al. Interleukin 17-producing $CD4^+$ effector T cells develop via a lineage distinct from the T helper type 1 and 2 lineages. Nature Immunology. 2005;**6**(11):1123-1132. DOI: 10.1038/ni1254

[47] Chizzolini C, Dufour AM, Brembilla NC. Is there a role for IL-17 in the pathogenesis of systemic sclerosis? Immunology Letters. 2018;**195**:61-67. DOI: 10.1016/j.imlet.2017.09.007

[48] Kolls JK, McCray PB Jr, Chan YR. Cytokine-mediated regulation of antimicrobial proteins. Nature Reviews. Immunology. 2008;**8**(11):829-835. DOI: 10.1038/nri2433

[49] Happel KI, Zheng M, Young E, Quinton LJ, Lockhart E, Ramsay AJ, et al. Cutting edge: Roles of toll-like receptor 4 and IL-23 in IL-17 expression in response to *Klebsiella pneumoniae* infection. Journal of Immunology. 2003;**170**(9):4432-4436. DOI: 10.4049/jimmunol.170.9.4432

[50] Ye P, Garvey PB, Zhang P, Nelson S, Bagby G, Summer WR, et al. Interleukin-17 and lung host defense against *Klebsiella pneumoniae* infection. American Journal of Respiratory Cell and Molecular Biology. 2001;**25**(3):335-340. DOI: 10.1165/ajrcmb.25.3.4424

[51] Chizzolini C, Chicheportiche R, Alvarez M, de Rham C, Roux-Lombard P, Ferrari-Lacraz S, et al. Prostaglandin E_2 synergistically with interleukin-23 favors human Th17 expansion. Blood. 2008;**112**(9):3696-3703. DOI: 10.1182/blood-2008-05-155408

[52] Dinarello CA, Novick D, Kim S, Kaplanski G. Interleukin-18 and IL-18 binding protein. Frontiers in Immunology. 2013;**4**:289. DOI: 10.3389/fimmu.2013.00289

[53] Murray HW. Interferon-γ and host antimicrobial defense: Current and future clinical applications. The American Journal of Medicine. 1994;**97**(5):459-467. DOI: 10.1016/0002-9343(94)90326-3

[54] Miettinen M, Matikainen S, Vuopio-Varkila J, Pirhonen J, Varkila K, Kurimoto M, et al. Lactobacilli and streptococci induced interleukin-12 (IL-12), IL-18, and gamma interferon production in human peripheral blood mononuclear cells. Infection and Immunity. 1998;**66**(12):6058-6062

[55] Antachopoulos C, Roilides E. Cytokines and fungal infections. British Journal of Haematology. 2005;**129**(5):583-596. DOI: 10.1111/j.1365-2141.2005.05498.x

[56] Hamad M. Innate and adaptive antifungal immune responses: Partners on an equal footing. Mycoses. 2012;**55**(3):205-217. DOI: 10.1111/j.1439-0507.2011.02078.x

[57] Mengesha BG, Conti HR. The role of IL-17 in protection against mucosal candida infections. Journal of Fungi. 2017;**3**(4):52-63. DOI: 10.3390/jof3040052

[58] Salazar F, Brown GD. Antifungal innate immunity: A perspective from the last 10 years. Journal of Innate Immunity. 2018;**16**:1-25. DOI: 10.1159/000488539

[59] Brown GD. Innate antifungal immunity: The key role of phagocytes. Annual Review of Immunology. 2011;**29**:1-21. DOI: 10.1146/annurev-immunol-030409-101229

[60] Verma A, Wüthrich M, Deepe G, Klein B. Adaptive immunity to fungi. Cold Spring Harbor Perspectives in Medicine. 2014;**5**(3):a019612-a019636. DOI: 10.1101/cshperspect.a019612

[61] Nadesalingam J, Dodds AW, Reid KB, Palaniyar N. Mannose-binding lectin recognizes peptidoglycan via the N-acetyl glucosamine moiety and inhibits ligand-induced proinflammatory effect and promotes chemokine production by macrophages. Journal of Immunology. 2005;**175**(3):1785-1794. DOI: 10.4049/jimmunol.175.3.1785

[62] Gafa V, Lande R, Gagliardi MC, Severa M, Giacomini E, Remoli ME, et al. Human dendritic cells following *Aspergillus fumigatus* infection express the CCR7 receptor and a differential

pattern of interleukin-12 (IL-12), IL-23, and IL-27 cytokines, which lead to a Th1 response. Infection and Immunity. 2006;**74**(3):1480-1489. DOI: 10.1128/IAI.74.3.1480-1489.2006

[63] Thompson A, Orr SJ. Emerging IL-12 family cytokines in the fight against fungal infections. Cytokine. 2018;**S1043-4666**(18):30218-30227. DOI: 10.1016/j.cyto.2018.05.019

[64] Balish E, Wagner RD, Vázquez-Torres A, Pierson C, Warner T. Candidiasis in interferon-gamma knockout (IFN-gamma−/−) mice. The Journal of Infectious Diseases. 1998;**178**(2):478-487. DOI: 10.1086/515645

[65] Hünniger K, Kurzai O. Phagocytes as central players in the defence against invasive fungal infection. Seminars in Cell & Developmental Biology. 2018;**S1084-9521**(17):30540-30552. DOI: 10.1016/j.semcdb.2018.03.021

[66] Conti HR, Shen F, Nayyar N, Stocum E, Sun JN, Lindemann MJ, et al. Th17 cells and IL-17 receptor signaling are essential for mucosal host defense against oral candidiasis. The Journal of Experimental Medicine. 2009;**206**(2):299-311. DOI: 10.1084/jem.20081463

[67] Oppmann B, Lesley B, Blom JC, Timans Y, Xu B, Hunte F, et al. Kastelein. Novel p19 protein engages IL-12p40 to form a cytokine: IL-23, with biological activities similar as well as distinct from IL-12. Immunity. 2000;**13**(5):715-725. DOI: 10.1016/S1074-7613(00)00070-4

[68] Mariangel A, Federica F, Daniela G, Silvia D, Silvio D. Can IL-23 be a good target for ulcerative colitis? Best Practice & Research. Clinical Gastroenterology. 2018;**32-33**:95-102. DOI: 10.1016/j.bpg.2018.05.016

[69] Huang W, Na L, Fidel PL, Schwarzenberger P. Requirement of interleukin-17A for systemic anti-Candida albicans host defense in mice. The Journal of Infectious Diseases. 2004;**190**(3):624-631. DOI: 10.1086/422329

[70] Mogensen TH, Paludan SR. Molecular pathways in virus-induced cytokine production. Microbiology and Molecular Biology Reviews. 2001;**65**(1):131-150. DOI: 10.1128/MMBR.65.1.131-150.2001

[71] Takeuchi O, Akira S. MDA5/RIG-I and virus recognition. Current Opinion in Immunology. 2008;**20**(1):17-22. DOI: 10.1016/j.coi.2008.01.002

[72] Barton GM. Viral recognition by Toll-like receptors. Seminars in Immunology. 2007;**19**(1):33-40. DOI: 10.1016/j.smim.2007.01.003

[73] Perrot I, Deauvieau F, Massacrier C, Hughes N, Garrone P, Durand I, et al. TLR3 and Rig-like receptor on myeloid dendritic cells and Rig-like receptor on human NK cells are both mandatory for production of IFN-gamma in response to double-stranded RNA. Journal of Immunology. 2010;**185**(4):2080-2088. DOI: 10.4049/jimmunol.1000532

[74] Kawai T, Akira S. Innate immune recognition of viral infection. Nature Immunology. 2006;**7**(2):131-137. DOI: 10.1038/ni1303

[75] Xagorari A, Chlichlia K. Toll-like receptors and viruses: Induction of innate antiviral immune responses. Open Microbiology Journal. 2008;**2**:49-59. DOI: 10.2174/1874285800802010049

[76] López S, Sánchez-Tacuba L, Moreno J, Arias CF. Rotavirus strategies against the innate antiviral system. Annual Review of Virology. 2016;**3**(1):591-609. DOI: 10.1146/annurev-virology-110615-042152

[77] Bixler SL, Goff AJ. The role of cytokines and chemokines in filovirus

infection. Viruses. 2015;**7**(10):5489-5507. DOI: 10.3390/v7102892

[78] Sennikov SV, Temchura VV, Trufakin VA, Kozlov VA. Effects of granulocyte-macrophage colony-stimulating factor produced by intestinal epithelial cells on functional activity of hemopoietic stem cells. Bulletin of Experimental Biology and Medicine. 2002;**134**(6):548-550. DOI: 10.1023/A:1022952810245

[79] Chan MC, Cheung CY, Chui WH, Tsao SW, Nicholls JM, Chan YO, et al. Proinflammatory cytokine responses induced by influenza A (H5N1) viruses in primary human alveolar and bronchial epithelial cells. Respiratory Research. 2005;**11**(6):135. DOI: 10.1186/1465-9921-6-135

[80] González-Amaro R, García-Monzón C, García-Buey L, Moreno-Otero R, Alonso JL, Yagüe E, et al. Induction of tumor necrosis factor alpha production by human hepatocytes in chronic viral hepatitis. Journal of Experimental Medicine. 1994;**179**(3):841-848

[81] Burbach GJ, Naik SM, Harten JB, Liu L, Dithmar S, Grossniklaus H, et al. Interleukin-18 expression and modulation in human corneal epithelial cells. Current Eye Research. 2001;**23**(1):64-68. DOI: 10.1076/ceyr.23.1.64.5425

[82] Walter MJ, Kajiwara N, Karanja P, Castro M, Holtzman MJ. Interleukin 12 p40 production by barrier epithelial cells during airway inflammation. Journal of Experimental Medicine. 2001;**193**(3):339-351

[83] Aoki Y, Qiu D, Uyei A, Kao PN. Human airway epithelial cells express interleukin-2 in vitro. The American Journal of Physiology. 1997;**272**(2 Pt 1):L276-L286. DOI: 10.1152/ajplung.1997.272.2.L276

[84] Piskin G, Sylva-Steenland RM, Bos JD, Teunissen MB. In vitro and in situ expression of IL-23 by keratinocytes in healthy skin and psoriasis lesions: Enhanced expression in psoriatic skin. Journal of Immunology. 2006;**176**(3):1908-1915. DOI: 10.4049/jimmunol.176.3.1908

[85] Yannam GR, Gutti T, Poluektova LY. IL-23 in infections, inflammation, autoimmunity and cancer: Possible role in HIV-1 and AIDS. Journal of Neuroimmune Pharmacology. 2012;**7**(1):95-112. DOI: 10.1007/s11481-011-9315-2

[86] Cotton JA, Platnich JM, Muruve DA, Jijon HB, Buret AG, Beck PL. Interleukin-8 in gastrointestinal inflammation and malignancy: Induction and clinical consequences. International Journal of Interferon and Cytokine Medical Research. 2016;**8**:13-34. DOI: 10.2147/IJICMR.S63682

[87] Hofmann P, Sprenger H, Kaufmann A, Bender A, Hasse C, Nain M, et al. Susceptibility of mononuclear phagocytes to influenza A virus infection and possible role in the antiviral response. Journal of Leukocyte Biology. 1997;**61**(4):408-414. DOI: 10.1002/jlb.61.4.408

[88] Nishitsuji H, Funami K, Shimizu Y, Ujino S, Sugiyama K, Seya T, et al. Hepatitis C virus infection induces inflammatory cytokines and chemokines mediated by the cross talk between hepatocytes and stellate cells. Journal of Virology. 2013;**87**(14):8169-8178. DOI: 10.1128/JVI.00974-13

[89] Jiang B, Snipes-Magaldi L, Dennehy P, Keyserling H, Holman RC, Bresee J, et al. Cytokines as mediators for or effectors against rotavirus disease in children. Clinical and Diagnostic Laboratory Immunology. 2003;**10**(6):995-1001. DOI: 10.1128/CDLI.10.6.995-1001.2003

[90] Hervas-Stubbs S, Perez-Gracia JL, Rouzaut A, Sanmamed MF, Le Bon A, Melero I. Direct effects of type I interferons on cells of the immune system. Clinical Cancer Research. 2011;**17**(9):2619-2627. DOI: 10.1158/1078-0432.CCR-10-1114

[91] Luft T, Pang KC, Thomas E, Hertzog P, Hart DN, Trapani J, et al. Type I IFNs enhance the terminal differentiation of dendritic cells. Journal of Immunology. 1998;**161**(4):1947-1953

[92] Le Bon A, Durand V, Kamphuis E, Thompson C, Bulfone-Paus S, Rossmann C, et al. Direct stimulation of T cells by type I IFN enhances the $CD8^+$ T cell response during cross-priming. Journal of Immunology. 2006;**176**(8):4682-4689. DOI: 10.4049/jimmunol.176.8.4682

[93] Freeman BE, Raué HP, Hill AB, Slifka MK. Cytokine-mediated activation of NK cells during viral infection. Journal of Virology. 2015;**89**(15):7922-7931. DOI: 10.1128/JVI.00199-15

[94] Ito H, Esashi E, Akiyama T, Inoue J, Miyajima A. IL-18 produced by thymic epithelial cells induces development of dendritic cells with CD11b in the fetal thymus. International Immunology. 2006;**18**(8):1253-1263. DOI: 10.1093/intimm/dxl058

[95] Striz I, Brabcova E, Kolesar L, Sekerkova A. Cytokine networking of innate immunity cells: A potential target of therapy. Clinical Science (London, England). 2014;**126**(9):593-612. DOI: 10.1042/CS20130497

[96] Seo SH, Webster RG. Tumor necrosis factor alpha exerts powerful anti-influenza virus effects in lung epithelial cells. Journal of Virology. 2002;**76**(3):1071-1076. DOI: 10.1128/JVI.76.3.1071-1076.2002

[97] Mosser DM, Edwards JP. Exploring the full spectrum of macrophage activation. Nature Reviews. Immunology. 2008;**8**(12):958-969. DOI: 10.1038/nri2448

[98] Eskilsson A, Mirrasekhian E, Dufour S, Schwaninger M, Engblom D, Blomqvist A. Immune-induced fever is mediated by IL-6 receptors on brain endothelial cells coupled to STAT3-dependent induction of brain endothelial prostaglandin synthesis. The Journal of Neuroscience. 2014;**34**(48):15957-15961. DOI: 10.1523/JNEUROSCI.3520-14.2014

[99] Di Paolo NC, Shayakhmetov DM. Interleukin 1α and the inflammatory process. Nature Immunology. 2016;**17**(8):906-913. DOI: 10.1038/ni.3503

[100] Opal SM, DePalo VA. Anti-inflammatory cytokines. Chest. 2000;**117**(4):1162-1172. DOI: 10.1378/chest.117.4.1162

[101] Reis C. Activation of dendritic cells: Translating innate into adaptive immunity. Current Opinion in Immunology. 2004;**16**(1):21-25. DOI: 10.1016/j.coi.2003.11.00

[102] Kapsenberg ML. Dendritic-cell control of pathogen-driven T-cell polarization. Nature Reviews. Immunology. 2003;**3**(12):984-993. DOI: 10.1038/nri1246

[103] Letterio JJ, Roberts AB. TGF-β: A critical modulator of immune cell function. Clinical Immunology and Immunopathology. 1997;**84**(3):244-250. DOI: 10.1006/clin.1997.4409

[104] Tanaka T, Narazaki M, Kishimoto T. IL-6 in inflammation, immunity, and disease. Cold Spring Harbor Perspectives in Biology. 2014;**6**(10):a016295. DOI: 10.1101/cshperspect.a016295

[105] Acosta-Rodriguez EV, Napolitani G, Lanzavecchia A, Sallusto F. Interleukins 1beta and 6 but not transforming growth factor-beta are essential for the differentiation of interleukin 17-producing human T helper cells. Nature Immunology. 2007;**8**(9):942-949. DOI: 10.1038/ni1496

[106] Friederichs K, Schmitz J, Weissenbach M, Heinrich PC, Schaper F. Interleukin-6-induced proliferation of pre-B cells mediated by receptor complexes lacking the SHP2/ SOCS3 recruitment sites revisited. European Journal of Biochemistry. 2001;**268**(24):6401-6407. DOI: 10.1046/j.0014-2956.2001.02586.x

[107] Ozaki K, Spolski R, Ettinger R, Kim HP, Wang G, Qi CF, et al. Regulation of B cell differentiation and plasma cell generation by IL-21, a novel inducer of Blimp-1 and Bcl-6. Journal of Immunology. 2004;**173**(9):5361-5371. DOI: 10.4049/jimmunol.173.9.5361

[108] Hilbert DM, Cancro MP, Scherle PA, Nordan RP, Van Snick J, Gerhard W, et al. T cell derived IL-6 is differentially required for antigen-specific antibody secretion by primary and secondary B cells. Journal of Immunology. 1989;**143**(12):4019-4024

[109] Placek K, Gasparian S, Coffre M, Maiella S, Sechet E, Bianchi E, et al. Integration of distinct intracellular signaling pathways at distal regulatory elements directs T-bet expression in human $CD4^+$ T cells. Journal of Immunology. 2009;**183**(12):7743-7751. DOI: 10.4049/jimmunol.0803812

[110] Schijns VE, Haagmans BL, Wierda CM, Kruithof B, Heijnen IA, Alber G, et al. Mice lacking IL-12 develop polarized Th1 cells during viral infection. Journal of Immunology. 1998;**160**(8):3958-3964

[111] Ansel KM, Djuretic I, Tanasa B, Rao A. Regulation of Th2 differentiation and Il4 locus accessibility. Annual Review of Immunology. 2006;**24**:607-656. DOI: 10.1146/annurev.immunol.23.021704.115821

[112] Cote-Sierra J, Foucras G, Guo L, Chiodetti L, Young HA, Hu-Li J, et al. Interleukin 2 plays a central role in Th2 differentiation. Proceedings of the National Academy of Sciences of the United States of America. 2004;**101**(11):3880-3885. DOI: 10.1073/pnas.0400339101

[113] Walker JA, McKenzie ANJ. TH2 cell development and function. Nature Reviews. Immunology. 2018;**18**(2):121-133. DOI: 10.1038/nri.2017.118

[114] Baecher-Allan C, Viglietta V, Hafler DA. Inhibition of human CD4(+)CD25(+high) regulatory T cell function. Journal of Immunology. 2002;**169**(11):6210-6217. DOI: 10.4049/jimmunol.169.11.6210

[115] Krausgruber T, Blazek K, Smallie T, Alzabin S, Lockstone H, Sahgal N, et al. IRF5 promotes inflammatory macrophage polarization and TH1-TH17 responses. Nature Immunology. 2011;**12**(3):231. DOI: 10.1038/ni.1990

[116] Willart MA, Deswarte K, Pouliot P, Braun H, Beyaert R, Lambrecht BN, et al. Interleukin-1α controls allergic sensitization to inhaled house dust mite via the epithelial release of GM-CSF and IL-33. The Journal of Experimental Medicine. 2012;**209**(8):1505-1517. DOI: 10.1084/jem.2011269

[117] Murray PR, Rosenthal KS, Pfaller MA, editors. Medical Microbiology. 9th ed. Elsevier Inc., Philadelphia, PA. 2015. 89 p. ISBN: 9780323299565

[118] Schnittger L, Florin-Christensen M. Introduction into parasitic protozoa. In: Florin-Christensen M, Schnittger L, editors. Parasitic Protozoa of Farm Animals and Pets. Switzerland: Springer

International Publishing; 2018. pp. 1-10 (Chapter 1). ISBN 978-3-319-70132-5

[119] Melby PC, Stephens R, Dann SM. Host defenses to protozoa. In: Rich RR, Fleisher TA, Shearer WT, Schroeder HW, Frew AJ, Weyand CM, editors. Clinical Immunology. 5th ed. London: Elsevier; 2019. pp. 425-435.e1. DOI: 10.1016/B978-0-7020-6896-6.00030-2

[120] Kumar H, Kawai T, Akira S. Pathogen recognition by the innate immune system. International Reviews of Immunology. 2011;**30**(1):16-34. DOI: 10.3109/08830185.2010.529976

[121] Li K, Qu S, Chen X, Wu Q, Shi M. Promising targets for cancer immunotherapy: TLRs, RLRs, and STING-mediated innate immune pathways. International Journal of Molecular Sciences. 2017;**18**(2):404. DOI: 10.3390/ijms18020404

[122] Muñoz-Carrillo JL, Ortega-Martín Del Campo J, Gutiérrez-Coronado O, Villalobos-Gutiérrez PT, Contreras-Cordero JF, Ventura-Juárez J. Adipose tissue and inflammation. In: Szablewski L, editor. Adipose Tissue. London: InTech; 2018. pp. 93-121. DOI: 10.5772/intechopen.74227

[123] Bansal D, Ave P, Kerneis S, Frileux P, Boché O, Baglin AC, et al. An ex-vivo human intestinal model to study *Entamoeba histolytica* pathogenesis. PLoS Neglected Tropical Diseases. 2009;**3**(11):e551. DOI: 10.1371/journal.pntd.0000551

[124] Galván-Moroyoqui JM, Del Carmen Domínguez-Robles M, Meza I. Pathogenic bacteria prime the induction of toll-like receptor signalling in human colonic cells by the Gal/GalNAc lectin carbohydrate recognition domain of *Entamoeba histolytica*. International Journal for Parasitology. 2011;**41**(10):1101-1112. DOI: 10.1016/j.ijpara.2011.06.003

[125] Sierra-Puente RE, Campos-Rodríguez R, Jarillo-Luna RA, Muñoz-Fernández L, Rodríguez MG, Muñoz-Ortega MH, et al. Expression of immune modulator cytokines in human fulminant amoebic colitis. Parasite Immunology. 2009;**31**(7):384-391. DOI: 10.1111/j.1365-3024.2009.01118.x

[126] Salata RA, Murray HW, Rubin BY, Ravdin JI. The role of gamma interferon in the generation of human macrophages cytotoxic for *Entamoeba histolytica* trophozoites. The American Journal of Tropical Medicine and Hygiene. 1987;**37**(1):72-78. DOI: 10.4269/ajtmh.1987.37.72

[127] Ghadirian E, Kongshavn PA. Activation of macrophages by *Entamoeba histolytica* extracts in mice. Microbial Pathogenesis. 1988;**5**(1):63-70. DOI: 10.1016/0882-4010(88)90082-4

[128] Denis M, Chadee K. Human neutrophils activated by interferon-gamma and tumour necrosis factor-alpha kill *Entamoeba histolytica* trophozoites in vitro. Journal of Leukocyte Biology. 1989;**46**(3):270-274. DOI: 10.1002/jlb.46.3.270

[129] Denis M, Chadee K. Cytokine activation of murine macrophages for in vitro killing of *Entamoeba histolytica* trophozoites. Infection and Immunity. 1989;**57**(6):1750-1756

[130] Ghadirian E, Denis M. In vivo activation of macrophages by IFN-γ to kill *Entamoeba histolytica* trophozoites in vitro. Parasite Immunology. 1992;**14**(4):397-404. DOI: 10.1111/j.1365-3024.1992.tb00014.x

[131] Lin JY, Chadee K. Macrophage cytotoxicity against *Entamoeba histolytica* trophozoites is mediated by nitric oxide from L-arginine. Journal of Immunology. 1992;**148**(12):3999-4005

[132] Espinosa-Cantellano M, Martínez-Palomo A. Pathogenesis of intestinal amebiasis: From molecules to disease. Clinical Microbiology Reviews. 2000;**13**(2):318-331. DOI: 10.1128/CMR.13.2.318-331.2000

[133] Guo X, Barroso L, Becker SM, Lyerly DM, Vedvick TS, Reed SG, et al. Protection against intestinal amebiasis by a recombinant vaccine is transferable by T cells and mediated by gamma interferon. Infection and Immunity. 2009;**77**(9):3909-3918. DOI: 10.1128/IAI.00487-09

[134] Sánchez-Guillén Mdel C, Pérez-Fuentes R, Salgado-Rosas H, Ruiz-Argüelles A, Ackers J, Shire A, et al. Differentiation of *Entamoeba histolytica/entamoeba* dispar by PCR and their correlation with humoral and cellular immunity in individuals with clinical variants of amoebiasis. The American Journal of Tropical Medicine and Hygiene. 2002;**66**(6):731-737

[135] Bansal D, Sehgal R, Chawla Y, Malla N, Mahajan RC. Cytokine mRNA expressions in symptomatic vs. asymptomatic amoebiasis patients. Parasite Immunology. 2005;**27**(1-2):37-43. DOI: 10.1111/j.1365-3024.2005.00739.x

[136] Seydel KB, Smith SJ, Stanley SL Jr. Innate immunity to amebic liver abscess is dependent on gamma interferon and nitric oxide in a murine model of disease. Infection and Immunity. 2000;**68**(1):400-402

[137] Houpt ER, Glembocki DJ, Obrig TG, Moskaluk CA, Lockhart LA, Wright RL, et al. The mouse model of amebic colitis reveals mouse strain susceptibility to infection and exacerbation of disease by CD4^{+} T cells. Journal of Immunology. 2002;**169**(8):4496-4503. DOI: 10.4049/jimmunol.169.8.4496

[138] Lin JY, Seguin R, Keller K, Chadee K. Transforming growth factor-beta 1 primes macrophages for enhanced expression of the nitric oxide synthase gene for nitric oxide-dependent cytotoxicity against *Entamoeba histolytica*. Immunology. 1995;**85**(3):400-407

[139] Seydel KB, Li E, Swanson PE, Stanley SL Jr. Human intestinal epithelial cells produce proinflammatory cytokines in response to infection in a SCID mouse-human intestinal xenograft model of amebiasis. Infection and Immunity. 1997;**65**(5):1631-1639

[140] Guo X, Stroup SE, Houpt E. Persistence of *Entamoeba histolytica* infection in CBA mice owes to intestinal IL-4 production and inhibition of protective IFN-gamma. Mucosal Immunology. 2008;**1**(2):139-146. DOI: 10.1038/mi.2007.1

[141] Babu S, Nutman TB. Immune responses to helminth infection. In: Rich RR, Fleisher TA, Shearer WT, Schroeder HW, Frew AJ, Weyand CM, editors. Clinical Immunology. 5th ed. London: Elsevier; 2019. pp. 437-447.e1. DOI: 10.1016/B978-0-7020-6896-6.00031-4

[142] Maizels RM, Hewitson JP, Smith KA. Susceptibility and immunity to helminth parasites. Current Opinion in Immunology. 2012;**24**(4):459-466. DOI: 10.1016/j.coi.2012.06.003

[143] Ilic N, Gruden-Movsesijan A, Sofronic-Milosavljevic L. *Trichinella spiralis*: Shaping the immune response. Immunologic Research. 2012;**52**(1-2):111-119. DOI: 10.1007/s12026-012-8287-5

[144] Ashour DS. *Trichinella spiralis* immunomodulation: An interactive multifactorial process. Expert Review of Clinical Immunology. 2013;**9**(7):669-675. DOI: 10.1586/1744666X.2013.811187

[145] Bruschi F, Chiumiento L. Immunomodulation in trichinellosis: Does *Trichinella* really escape the host immune system? Endocrine, Metabolic & Immune Disorders Drug Targets. 2012;**12**(1):4-15. DOI: 10.2174/187153012799279081

[146] Cieza RJ, Cao AT, Cong Y, Torres AG. 2012. Immunomodulation for gastrointestinal infections. Expert Review of Anti-Infective Therapy. 2012;**10**(3):391-400. DOI: 10.1586/eri.11.176

[147] Ilic N, Worthington JJ, Gruden-Movsesijan A, Travis MA, Sofronic-Milosavljevic L, Grencis RK. *Trichinella spiralis* antigens prime mixed Th1/Th2 response but do not induce de novo generation of Foxp3⁺ T cells in vitro. Parasite Immunology. 2011;**33**(10):572-582. DOI: 10.1111/j.1365-3024.2011.01322.x

[148] Sofronic-Milosavljevic L, Ilic N, Pinelli E, Gruden-Movsesijan A. Secretory products of *Trichinella spiralis* muscle larvae and immunomodulation: Implication for autoimmune diseases, allergies, and malignancies. Journal of Immunology Research. 2015;**2015**:523875. DOI: 10.1155/2015/523875

[149] Gruden-Movsesijan A, Ilic N, Colic M, Majstorovic I, Vasilev S, Radovic I, et al. The impact of *Trichinella spiralis* excretory-secretory products on dendritic cells. Comparative Immunology, Microbiology and Infectious Diseases. 2011;**34**(5):429-439. DOI: 10.1016/j.cimid.2011.08.004

[150] Gentilini MV, Nuñez GG, Roux ME, Venturiello SM. *Trichinella spiralis* infection rapidly induces lung inflammatory response: The lung as the site of helminthocytotoxic activity. Immunobiology. 2011;**216**(9):1054-1063. DOI: 10.1016/j.imbio.2011.02.002

[151] Yu YR, Deng MJ, Lu WW, Jia MZ, Wu W, Qi YF. Systemic cytokine profiles and splenic toll-like receptor expression during *Trichinella spiralis* infection. Experimental Parasitology. 2013;**134**(1):92-101. DOI: 10.1016/j.exppara.2013.02.014

[152] Muñoz-Carrillo JL, Contreras-Cordero JF, Muñoz-López JL, Maldonado-Tapia CH, Muñoz-Escobedo JJ, Moreno-García MA. Resiniferatoxin modulates the Th1 immune response and protects the host during intestinal nematode infection. Parasite Immunology. 2017;**39**(9):1-16. DOI: 10.1111/pim.12448

[153] Ilic N, Colic M, Gruden-Movsesijan A, Majstorovic I, Vasilev S, Sofronic-Milosavljevic LJ. Characterization of rat bone marrow dendritic cells initially primed by *Trichinella spiralis* antigens. Parasite Immunology. 2008;**30**(9):491-495. DOI: 10.1111/j.1365-3024.2008.01049.x

[154] Ming L, Peng RY, Zhang L, Zhang CL, Lv P, Wang ZQ, et al. Invasion by *Trichinella spiralis* infective larvae affects the levels of inflammatory cytokines in intestinal epithelial cells in vitro. Experimental Parasitology. 2016;**170**:220-226. DOI: 10.1016/j.exppara.2016.10.003

[155] Muñoz-Carrillo JL, Muñoz-Escobedo JJ, Maldonado-Tapia CH, Chávez-Ruvalcaba F, Moreno-García MA. Resiniferatoxin lowers TNF-α, NO and PGE_2 in the intestinal phase and the parasite burden in the muscular phase of *Trichinella spiralis* infection. Parasite Immunology. 2017;**39**(1):1-14. DOI: 10.1111/pim.12393

[156] Helmby H, Grencis RK. IFN-gamma-independent effects of IL-12 during intestinal nematode infection. Journal of Immunology.

2003;**171**(7):3691-3696. DOI: 10.4049/jimmunol.171.7.3691

[157] Mühl H, Pfeilschifter J. Anti-inflammatory properties of pro-inflammatory interferon-gamma. International Immunopharmacology. 2003;**3**(9):1247-1255. DOI: 10.1016/S1567-5769(03)00131-0

[158] Neumann B, Emmanuilidis K, Stadler M, Holzmann B. Distinct functions of interferon-gamma for chemokine expression in models of acute lung inflammation. Immunology. 1998;**95**(4):512-521. DOI: 10.1046/j.1365-2567.1998.00643.x

[159] Roy A, Sawesi O, Pettersson U, Dagälv A, Kjellén L, Lundén A, et al. Serglycin proteoglycans limit enteropathy in *Trichinella spiralis*-infected mice. BMC Immunology. 2016;**17**(1):15. DOI: 10.1186/s12865-016-0155-y

[160] Ierna MX, Scales HE, Müller C, Lawrence CE. 2009. Transmembrane tumor necrosis factor alpha is required for enteropathy and is sufficient to promote parasite expulsion in gastrointestinal helminth infection. Infection and Immunity. 2009;**77**(9):3879-3885. DOI: 10.1128/IAI.01461-08

[161] Lawrence CE, Paterson J, Higgins LM, MacDonald TT, Kennedy MW, Garside P. IL-4-regulated enteropathy in an intestinal nematode infection. European Journal of Immunology. 1998;**28**(9):2672-2684. DOI: 10.1002/(SICI)1521-4141(199809)28:09<2672::AID-IMMU2672>3.0.CO;2-F

[162] Ierna MX, Scales HE, Saunders KL, Lawrence CE. Mast cell production of IL-4 and TNF may be required for protective and pathological responses in gastrointestinal helminth infection. Mucosal Immunology. 2008;**1**(2):147-155. DOI: 10.1038/mi.2007.16

[163] Bogdan C. Nitric oxide and the immune response. Nature Immunology. 2001;**2**(10):907-916. DOI: 10.1038/ni1001-907

[164] Guzik TJ, Korbut R, Adamek-Guzik T. Nitric oxide and superoxide in inflammation and immune regulation. Journal of Physiology and Pharmacology. 2003;**54**(4):469-487

[165] Wink DA, Hines HB, Cheng RYS, Switzer CH, Flores-Santana W, Vitek MP, et al. Nitric oxide and redox mechanisms in the immune response. Journal of Leukocyte Biology. 2011;**89**(6):873-891. DOI: 10.1189/jlb.1010550

[166] Andrade MA, Siles-Lucas M, López-Abán J, Nogal-Ruiz JJ, Pérez-Arellano JL, Martínez-Fernández AR, et al. Trichinella: Differing effects of antigens from encapsulated and non-encapsulated species on in vitro nitric oxide production. Veterinary Parasitology. 2007;**143**(1):86-90. DOI: 10.1016/j.vetpar.2006.07.026

[167] Moncada S, Erusalimsky JD. Does nitric oxide modulate mitochondrial energy generation and apoptosis? Nature Reviews. Molecular Cell Biology. 2002;**3**(3):214-220. DOI: 10.1038/nrm762

[168] Lawrence CE, Paterson JC, Wei XQ, Liew FY, Garside P, Kennedy MW. Nitric oxide mediates intestinal pathology but not immune expulsion during *Trichinella spiralis* infection in mice. Journal of Immunology. 2000;**164**(8):4229-4234. DOI: 10.4049/jimmunol.164.8.4229

[169] Cvetkovic J, Sofronic-Milosavljevic L, Ilic N, Gnjatovic M, Nagano I, Gruden-Movsesijan A.

Immunomodulatory potential of particular *Trichinella spiralis* muscle larvae excretory-secretory components. International Journal for Parasitology. 2016;**46**(13-14):833-842. DOI: 10.1016/j.ijpara.2016.07.008

[170] Ding J, Bai X, Wang X, Shi H, Cai X, Luo X, et al. Immune cell responses and cytokine profile in intestines of mice infected with *Trichinella spiralis*. Frontiers in Microbiology. 2017;**8**:2069. DOI: 10.3389/fmicb.2017.02069

[171] Helmby H, Grencis RK. Contrasting roles for IL-10 in protective immunity to different life cycle stages of intestinal nematode parasites. European Journal of Immunology. 2003;**33**(9):2382-2390. DOI: 10.1002/eji.200324082

[172] Urban JF, Schopf L, Morris SC, Orekhova T, Madden KB, Betts CJ, et al. Stat6 signaling promotes protective immunity against *Trichinella spiralis* through a mast cell-and T cell-dependent mechanism. Journal of Immunology. 2000;**164**(4):2046-2052. DOI: 10.4049/jimmunol.164.4.2046

[173] Akiho H, Blennerhassett P, Deng Y, Collins SM. Role of IL-4, IL-13, and STAT6 in inflammation-induced hypercontractility of murine smooth muscle cells. American Journal of Physiology. Gastrointestinal and Liver Physiology. 2002;**282**(2):G226-G232. DOI: 10.1152/ajpgi.2002.282.2.G226

[174] Scales HE, Ierna MX, Lawrence CE. The role of IL-4, IL-13 and IL-4Ralpha in the development of protective and pathological responses to *Trichinella spiralis*. Parasite Immunology. 2007;**29**(2):81-91. DOI: 10.1111/j.1365-3024.2006.00920.x

[175] Gurish MF, Bryce PJ, Tao H, Kisselgof AB, Thornton EM, Miller HR, et al. IgE enhances parasite clearance and regulates mast cell responses in mice infected with *Trichinella spiralis*. Journal of Immunology. 2004;**172**(2):1139-1145. DOI: 10.4049/jimmunol.172.2.1139

[176] Yasuda K, Nakanishi K. Host responses to intestinal nematodes. International Immunology. 2018;**30**(3):93-102. DOI: 10.1093/intimm/dxy002

[177] Wang LJ, Cao Y, Shi HN. Helminth infections and intestinal inflammation. World Journal of Gastroenterology. 2008;**14**:5125-5132

[178] Muñoz-Carrillo JL, Muñoz-López JL, Muñoz-Escobedo JJ, Maldonado-Tapia C, Gutiérrez-Coronado O, Contreras-Cordero JF, et al. Therapeutic effects of resiniferatoxin related with immunological responses for intestinal inflammation in trichinellosis. The Korean Journal of Parasitology. 2017;**55**(6):587-599. DOI: 10.3347/kjp.2017.55.6.587

Chapter 3

Nucleated Red Blood Cells Contribute to the Host Immune Response Against Pathogens

Verónica Chico, Ivan Nombela, Sara Puente-Marín and María del Mar Ortega-Villaizan

Abstract

It has recently come to light that nucleated red blood cells (RBCs) of fish, amphibians, reptiles and birds are multifunctional cells, because in addition to being involved in gas exchange and transport, it has also been reported that they respond to pathogens by means of (i) phagocytosis, (ii) antigen presentation, (iii) production of cytokines and antimicrobial peptides, (iv) regulation of complement system, and (v) exerting paracrine molecular communication with other immune cells and modulating their functions. Similarly, human cord blood nucleated RBCs have been shown to exert a regulatory function in the innate immune response, by means of the suppression of the production of inflammatory cytokines. This chapter comprises the study of the implications of nucleated RBCs as mediators of both branches of immune system (innate and adaptive immune responses).

Keywords: nucleated red blood cells, erythrocytes, immune response, cytokines, antimicrobial peptides, virus, antigen presentation

1. Introduction

Red blood cells (RBCs) are the most abundant cell type in the bloodstream, and their life span has been estimated to be 120 and 50 days in human and murine species, respectively [1]. In mammals, mature RBCs are biconcave disks that lack cell nucleus, organelles, and ribosomes [2], and their best known function is gas exchange and respiration. However, the most characteristic feature of nonmammalian RBCs is the presence of a nucleus which allows them to transcribe and translate proteins and therefore intervene in additional functions different from delivery of oxygen to tissues (**Figure 1**) [3]. The nucleated RBCs are able to respond against pathogens by employing various mechanisms. This chapter review encompasses the up-to-date studies about the involvement of nucleated red blood cells (RBCs) as immune response cell mediators against microbes.

2. The role of nucleated RBCs in innate immune system

The innate immune system is an evolutionarily older defense strategy found in many organisms such as animals, plants, fungi, insects, and primitive multicellular

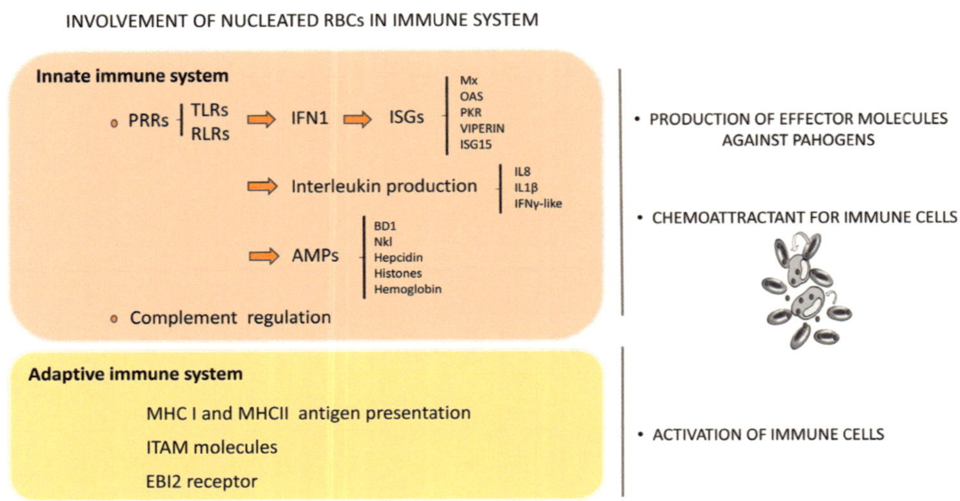

Figure 1.
Schematic representation of the suggested roles of nucleated RBCs in the immune response. *PRRs, pattern recognition receptors; TLRs, Toll-like receptor; RLR, RIG-I like receptor; IFN1, interferon type 1; ISGs, interferon-stimulated genes; Mx, myxovirus resistance gene; OAS, oligoadenylate synthetase; PKR, protein kinase RNA-activated; ISG15, interferon-stimulated gene 15; IL8, interleukin 8; IL1β, interleukin 1β; IFNγ-like, interferon γ-like; AMPs, antimicrobial peptides; BD1, β-defensin; Nkl, Nk-lysin; MHC, major histocompatibility complex; ITAM, immunoreceptor tyrosine-based activation motif; and EBI2, Epstein–Barr virus G-protein-coupled receptor 2.*

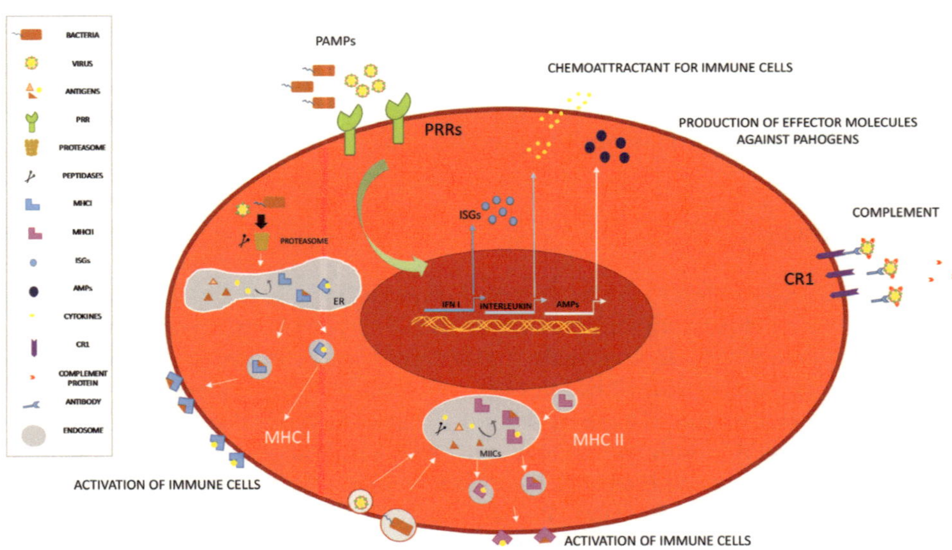

Figure 2.
Nucleated RBCs immune response suggested signaling involved in production of effector molecules against pathogens, chemoattractant proteins, and activation of immune cells. *PAMPs from microbes are recognized by specific PRRs. Activation of these receptors triggers the signaling pathways that induce the transcription of a set of genes such as IFN1, ISGs, interleukins, and AMPs. On the other hand, pathogens can be recognized by proteasome proteins and digested by peptidases. In the endoplasmic reticulum (ER), digested antigens from proteasome are bound to MHCI and exposed on the surface of RBCs. In addition, pathogens can enter inside the cell by endocytosis and delivered to MHC class II-loading compartments (MIICs) where they are digested and finally exposed on the surface of the cells by MHC II complex. Another pathway is the recognition of complement-opsonized immune complexes by CR1.*

organisms. This system is the first line of defense against pathogen infections. It is known as non-specific immune system and does not provide long-lasting immunity to the host [4, 5]. The innate immune system includes many types of molecules (receptors and effectors) to sense and eliminate pathogens. Moreover, nucleated RBCs release signaling molecules that trigger the activation of adaptive immune system. The implication of these cells in the innate immune response described to date is shown in **Figures 1** and **2**.

2.1 Nucleated RBCs trigger IFN type I response

It has been reported that nucleated RBCs do express pattern recognition receptors (PRRs) for pathogen-associated molecular patterns (PAMPs) [6]. PAMPs are small molecular motifs conserved in evolution and characteristic from pathogens. There are a vast variety of PAMPs, for example, bacterial lipopolysaccharides (LPS), bacterial flagellin, lipoteichoic acid from Gram-positive bacteria, peptidoglycan, and nucleic acid variants from viruses—such as double-stranded RNA (dsRNA) or nonmethylated viral 5'-C-phosphate-G-3′ (CpG)-containing DNA [7, 8]. PAMPs are recognized by the host cells through their PRRs such as Toll-like receptors (TLRs), retinoid acid-inducible gene I (RIG-I)-like receptors (RLRs), AIM2-like receptors (ALRs), and nucleotide-binding oligomerization domain (NOD)-like receptors (NLRs) [8, 9].

Among these receptors, a wide repertoire of TLRs have been described in nucleated RBCs, which allow them to respond to both bacterial and viral pathogens [10]. Chicken RBCs constitutively express gene transcripts of *tlr3* (which recognize viral patterns like viral double-stranded RNA (dsRNA)), *tlr21* (a homolog of mammalian TLR9 [3, 10]), and *tlr2*, *tlr4*, and *tlr5* (which recognize bacterial patterns [10]). In addition, rainbow trout RBCs [3, 11] and Atlantic salmon RBCs [12] constitutively express genes *tlr3* and *tlr9*, which recognizes CpG motifs present in microbial genome. Besides, *tlr3* upregulation with polyinosinic:polycytidylic acid (polyI:C, a molecule structurally similar to dsRNA) was found in tilapia RBCs [13]. It is noteworthy to highlight that it has been reported that the type of TLRs found in chicken nucleated RBCs is equivalent to that of many types of leukocytes [14]. This could be due to the fact that chicken RBCs and myeloid cells arise from a common progenitor cell [15].

Among RLRs, a family of receptors which interact intracellularly with viral dsRNA [3, 11, 12], RIG-I has also been reported in salmon RBCs. However, the expression of other members of RLR family, such as melanoma differentiation-associated protein 5 (MDA5) or probable ATP-dependent RNA helicase DExH-box helicase 58 (LGP2), in nucleated RBCs is still unknown [16].

Activation of these receptors with their corresponding PAMPs triggers the signaling networks that induce the transcription of a set of genes characteristic of the innate immune response such as the expression of interferon type I (IFN1) [17, 18]. The IFN1 is reportedly known to play a similar role in mammalian and nonmammalian species [19]. The binding of IFN1 to their cellular receptors induces different cell signaling pathways leading to the transcription of interferon-stimulated genes (ISGs), including important mediators of antiviral response such as myxovirus resistance protein (Mx), 2′–5′oligoadenylate synthetase (OAS), protein kinase RNA-activated (PKR), viperin, interferon-stimulated gene 15 (ISG15), IFN-induced protein with tetratricopeptide repeats (IFIT), and tripartite motif (TRIM) family, tetherin, among others [20].

In this regard, chicken and rainbow trout RBCs treated with polyI:C have been reported to induce upregulation of type I IFNs [3, 10] and also interferon-inducible genes Mx [3] and OAS [10], a protein responsible for initiating the RNAse L pathway in order to cleave viral RNA [21]. In addition, it has been described that nucleated RBCs when infected with a virus increase the expression of IFN1 and their ISGs. A study of Atlantic salmon-infected individuals with salmon anemia virus (ISAV) first demonstrated the ability of RBCs to induce *ifnα* expression in hemagglutinated RBCs [22]. In another example, Atlantic salmon challenged with piscine orthoreovirus (PRV), PRV-infected RBCs, induced the expression of *ifn1*, *mx*, *pkr* [23], *viperin*, and *isg15* [24] antiviral genes. Recently, Nombela and colleagues demonstrated that rainbow trout RBCs could generate IFN1-related responses to viruses despite not being infected. In response to infectious pancreatic necrosis virus (IPNV), authors observed that ex vivo purified RBCs exposed to the virus showed an increment in the expression of *ifn1*, *mx*, interferon regulatory factor7 (*irf7*), and *pkr* genes followed by upregulation of Mx protein expression [25]. Likely to IPNV, viral hemorrhagic septicemia virus (VHSV) was unable to replicate in ex vivo purified rainbow trout RBCs [26]. However, rainbow trout RBCs exposed to this virus showed a decrease in the expression of genes related to IFN1 pathway. The possible explanation that the authors found for this phenomenon was a process characterized by global proteome downregulation or shutoff in order to inhibit viral protein synthesis [26]. In addition, high levels of constitutive Mx transcripts and protein were also identified in rainbow trout RBCs (**Figure 3**) suggesting that the expression of this ISG could be a possible mechanism for aborted or halted infections in rainbow trout RBCs [25, 26].

Nevertheless, the involvement of IFN 1 response in nucleated RBCs and how does this response influence the global defense against viral infections remain to be demonstrated.

2.2 Nucleated RBCs induce interleukin response

TLR signaling culminates in cellular activation and production of cytokines [27]. Cytokines are secreted proteins involved in cell recruitment and regulation of both innate and adaptive immune responses. They are essential for an effective host immune response to pathogens [28]. The nucleated RBCs apart from type I IFN expression have been reported to produce other cytokines, at gene or protein level, in response to several PAMPs.

Chicken RBCs stimulated with polyI:C have shown an increase in interleukin 8 (*il8*) transcripts of approximately 4 log, which was at least two to three orders of

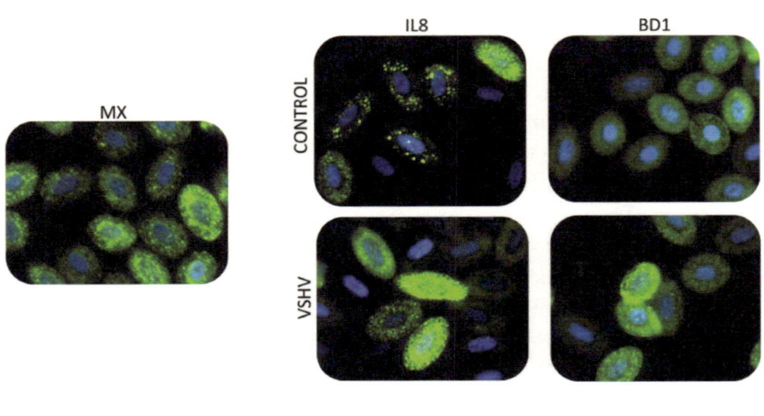

Figure 3.
Representative innate immune response in rainbow trout RBCs. *Representative immunofluorescence of Mx constitutive expression in rainbow trout RBCs. Representative immunofluorescence of IL8 and BD1 protein expression in rainbow trout RBCs control and exposed to VHSV. Images were taken using INCell Analyzer 6000 Cell imaging system (GE Healthcare, Little Chalfont, United Kingdom). FITC, fluorescein-5-isothiocyanate—for protein stain; DAPI, 4′,6-diamidino-2-phenylindole—for nuclei stain; Mx, myxovirus resistance protein; IL8, interleukin 8; BD1, β-defensin 1; and RBC, red blood cells.*

magnitude higher than those observed in monocytes, thrombocytes, and heterophils [10]. Besides, stimulation of rainbow trout RBCs with polyI:C was reported to induce de novo synthesis of mRNAs from chemokine (C-C motif) ligand 4 (*ccl4*) [3], which is a chemoattractant for natural killer cells, monocytes, and a variety of other immune cells [29].

Rainbow trout RBCs exposed to VHSV have shown augmented IL-8 (**Figure 3**) and interleukin 1β (IL-1β) protein levels [26]. IL-8 acts as a chemotactic factor for heterophils and other leukocytes such as monocytes [30]. Further studies are needed to consider the chemotactic properties of nucleated RBCs, however. On the other hand, rainbow trout RBCs exposed to IPNV showed a downregulation trend of IL-8, IL-1β, and tumor necrosis factor-α (TNF-α) protein expression [25]. Similarly, human cord blood nucleated RBCs have been shown to exert a regulatory function in the innate immune response, by means of the suppression of the production of inflammatory cytokines such as TNF-α and IL-1β from monocytes in lipopolysaccharide (LPS)-mimicked system to suppress a vigorous innate immune reaction, which can be harmful to fetuses [31].

Interferon gamma (IFNγ), a highly pleiotropic pro-inflammatory and antiviral cytokine exclusively produced in immune-related cells, has been detected in murine nucleated erythroid cells and may exert a regulatory influence on development and functionality of cells pertaining to monocyte/ macrophage lineage [32]. In addition, it has been shown that chicken RBCs stimulated with fungal species *Candida albicans* release cytokine-like factors with IFNγ-like activity [33]. The conditioned medium of shape-shifted RBCs (shRBCs), a new cell stage of rainbow trout RBCs, induced communication with rainbow trout stromal pronephros cells (TPS-2 cells) and resulted in the upregulation of IFNγ-activated genes in this cell line [34].

Taken altogether, these evidences indicate that nucleated RBCs exert paracrine molecular communication with other cells by means of cytokine production. Therefore, nucleated RBCs could play an important role in the recruitment and/or activation of immune cells.

2.3 Nucleated RBCs produce antimicrobial peptide and protein expression

Antimicrobial peptides (AMPs) exist in all living creatures in nature and present the first line of host defense against infectious pathogens [35] by means of molecular mechanisms of cellular disruption [36] and multifaceted immunomodulatory functions [35]. Fish nucleated RBCs have been reported to produce antimicrobial peptides in response to the viral infection.

Rainbow trout RBCs expose to VHSV induced an upregulation of β-defensin 1 (BD1) protein levels (**Figure 3**). Defensins belong to a family of small cysteine-rich peptides that have amphiphilic and cationic properties [37]. BD is produced and stored in epithelial cells, neutrophils, and phagocytes [38]. During infection by pathogens, BD stored in granular bodies is released into the phagosomes or the extracellular system [38]. Additionally, they are known as chemotactic attractants for immune cells and participate in immune regulation [39].

Another AMP recently found in fish RBCs is Nk-lysin (Nkl) [40]. Nkl is orthologous to human cytolytic protein granulysin, produced by natural killer cells and cytotoxic T lymphocytes [41, 42], and involved in the destruction of bacteria, fungi, and parasites [43]. Nkl is stored in cytolytic granules together with perforin and granzymes [41, 42]. However, Nkl in turbot RBCs was found in autophagolysosomes. This is reportedly known to link mechanism to VHSV defense in turbot RBCs [40].

Hepcidins, another family of cysteine-rich antimicrobial peptides, have also been found to be produced by fish RBCs [26]. They were first identified in the human liver [44] and also in some fish species [45]. But these peptides have also been reported to be expressed in other organs such as cardiac stomach, esophagus [46], heart, gill, spleen, kidney, and peripheral blood leucocytes [47] dependent upon the species. They have been shown to respond to bacterial and viral infections [48]. Regarding RBCs, Nombela and colleagues found that rainbow trout RBCs exposed to VHSV did not vary hepcidin protein levels [26]. Therefore, the possible role of hepcidin in nucleated RBCs against infectious pathogens is not known yet.

Histone proteins share all of the essential traits of cationic AMPs (CAMPs); they are hydrophobic and cationic and can form amphipathic alpha-helical structures [49]. Recently, it has been demonstrated that a histone mixture (H1, H2A, H2B, H3, H4, and H5) extracted and purified from chicken RBCs had antimicrobial activity against a variety of Gram-negative and Gram-positive planktonic bacteria [50], as well as eradication activity against Gram-positive bacterial biofilms [51]. It has also been reported that histone H5 from chicken RBCs has a broad-spectrum antimicrobial activity [52].

In addition to AMPs, another protein with antimicrobial activity found in RBCs is hemoglobin [53], which is the most abundant protein of RBCs. It has been described that hemoglobin can elicit antimicrobial activity through reactive oxygen species production under pathogen attack [53]. The pathogen clearance from the bloodstream is also carried out by the hemoglobin oxygen [54].

In brief, nucleated RBCs can produce antimicrobial molecules in response to pathogens. It therefore supports the important contribution of RBCs in the regulation of host defense against pathogens.

2.4 Complement regulation on RBCs

The complement system is a component of the innate immune system which is involved in the clearance of pathogens, dying cells and immune complexes through opsonization, induction of an inflammatory response, and formation of a lytic pore. This system is composed by a group of 30 different plasma and membrane proteins, which are involved in three distinct pathways of complement activation: the classical, lectin, and alternative pathway. The classical pathway is activated by immune complexes, by pattern recognition molecules such as C-reactive protein (CRP), or directly by apoptotic cells and microbial surfaces. The lectin pathway is triggered by carbohydrate structures from pathogen, and the alternative pathway is activated by the spontaneous hydrolysis of the protein C3 (reviewed in [55]).

Autologous cells are protected from complement activation and posterior lysis by regulatory proteins [56]. RBCs are continuously in contact with complement proteins in the blood plasma; therefore, they have complement regulatory proteins on their cell membrane to prevent this activation [55]. It has been reported that human and rainbow trout RBCs highly express the regulatory protein complement receptor 1 (CR1) or CD35 [56, 57]. An important function of RBC CR1 is to eliminate complement-opsonized immune complexes from the circulation. A failure in this receptor can end up in inflammation and damage to healthy tissues [58]. In addition, it has been described that human RBCs can sequester typ. 5 adenovirus (Ad5) through CR1 and Coxsackie virus-adenovirus receptor (CAR), in the presence and absence of anti-Ad5 antibodies and complement, respectively. In this context, human RBCs may act as circulating viral traps or clarifiers and prevent systemic virus infection [59]. The studies of immune complex clearance in rainbow trout showed a similar complement-dependent way to eliminate immune complex as found in humans, suggesting that rainbow trout CR1 has a similar function to human CR1 [60].

3. The role of nucleated RBCs in adaptive immune response activation

The adaptive immune system consists of a specialized group of cells responsible of a specific immune response which eliminates and prevents reoccurrence of pathogens by immunological memory [61]. The cells that carry out adaptive immune response are B and T lymphocytes [62]. All nucleated cells are capable of presenting an antigen, through major histocompatibility complex (MHC) molecules [62]. MHCI plays a key role in antigen presentation of intracellular pathogens. Nucleated RBCs can express MHCI, and this molecule has been found on the surface of RBCs from rainbow trout [63], African clawed frogs [64], and chickens [65]. In addition, it has been reported that PRV infection induces genes involved in antigen presentation via MHCI in salmon RBCs [23], and incubation with polyI:C upregulates gene ontology (GO) categories related to antigen processing, antigen presentation, and MHCI receptor activity in rainbow trout RBCs [6]. Unlike MHCI, MHCII molecules are generally restricted to some endothelial cells and a subset of antigen-presenting cells (APCs), such as macrophages, dendritic cells, and B cells [66]. However, MHCII transcripts have been detected in chicken [10] and rainbow trout RBCs [67]. Moreover, in rainbow trout RBCs, a combination of transcriptome- and proteome-sequencing data identified functional pathways related to antigen presentation via major histocompatibility complex class II. The set of genes/proteins identified were ARP1 actin-related protein 1 homolog B (ACTR1B), adaptor-related protein complex 1 beta 1 subunit (AP1B1), adaptor-related protein complex 2 alpha 1 subunit (AP2A1), adaptor-related protein complex 2 alpha 2 subunit (AP2A2), ADP ribosylation factor 1 (ARF1), calnexin (CANX), capping actin protein of muscle Z-line alpha subunit 1 (CAPZA1), clathrin light chain A (CLTA), clathrin heavy chain (CLTC), cathepsin D (CTSD), dynamin 2 (DNM2), dynein cytoplasmic 1 heavy chain 1 (DYNC1H1), dynein light chain LC8 typ. 2 (DYNLL2), and member RAS oncogene family (RAB7A) (**Figure 4**) [67].

Taking the above-said observations into account, these facts indicate that nucleated RBCs might participate in antigen presentation through MHCI and MHCII and suggest that RBCs may be participants in the immunological synapse with T and NK cells. Besides, it has been published that human RBCs could play a biological role in the modulation of T-cell differentiation and survival in the active cell division [68]. Also, natural killer enhancing factor (NKEF) protein in human RBC cytosol mediates enhancement of NK cell activity [69]. In addition, in rainbow trout RBCs, functional pathways related to regulation of leukocyte activation were identified by a combination of transcriptome- and proteome-sequencing data [67]. Separately, rainbow trout RBCs have been reported to use phagocytosis to bind and engulf *Candida albicans* and present it to macrophages [70]. In fact, the identification of clusters of cells composed by RBCs and immune cells, commonly termed rosettes, leads to a crosstalk between RBCs and immune cells [70]. These evidences broaden the horizon of nucleated RBC immune functions as they open a novel topic of investigation where nucleated RBCs may act as professional APCs.

Separately, other molecules related to adaptive immune response have been identified in nucleated RBCs. An example of these molecules is the immunoreceptor tyrosine-based activation motif (ITAM) which is contained in certain transmembrane proteins of the immune system and is important for the signal transduction in immune cells [71]. ITAM-bearing molecules are expressed on rainbow trout RBCs [72]. Another molecule, Epstein–Barr virus G-protein-coupled receptor 2 (EBI2), which plays a critical role in the regulation of T-cell-dependent antibody responses and provides a mechanism to balance short- versus long-term antibody responses [73], has also been reported to be highly expressed in rainbow trout young RBCs

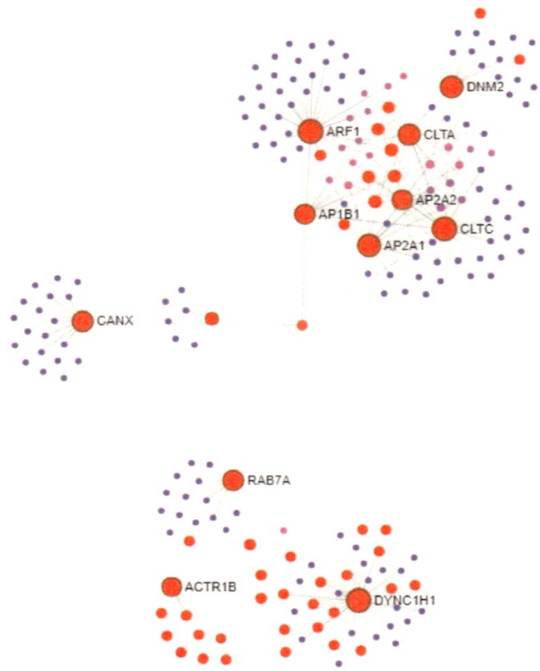

Figure 4.
An overview of protein–protein interaction network of a set of proteins, identified in rainbow trout proteome profiling, related to antigen processing and presentation of exogenous peptide antigen via MHCII. *Protein–protein interaction network was constructed using NetworkAnalyst software [75]. Highlighted red nodes represent the input protein-related antigen processing and presentation of exogenous peptide antigen via MHCII pathway (Reactome database). Other nodes represent other protein interactions within the same pathway (red nodes) or related to other pathways (other colors).*

[74]. Based on these facts, a role for RBCs in the adaptive immune response may be established. However, the function of these molecules and their effect on the antiviral adaptive immune response of nucleated RBCs remain to be studied.

4. Conclusion

Nucleated red blood cells (RBCs) of fish, amphibians, reptiles, and birds contain the transcriptional and translational machinery necessary to produce characteristic molecules of the immune system to respond against pathogen attacks. The mechanisms by which nucleated RBCs may contribute to the clearance of the pathogens are (i) phagocytosis, (ii) antigen presentation, (iii) producing cytokines and antimicrobial peptides, (iv) regulation of complement system, and (v) exerting paracrine molecular communication with other immune cells and modulate their functions. The nucleated RBCs seem to be involved in regulation of both innate and adaptive immune responses, and these findings highlight the important contribution of RBCs in the host defense against pathogens. However, more studies are needed to elucidate the role of RBCs in the immune response and the molecular mechanisms involved in these processes. And, the RBCs could be considered as potential targets for new prophylactic or therapeutic strategies against viral infections.

Acknowledgements

This work was supported by the European Research Council (ERC Starting Grant GA639249). The authors would like to thank Remedios Torres and Efren Lucas for their technical assistance.

Conflict of interest

The authors declare no conflict of interest.

Author details

Verónica Chico, Ivan Nombela, Sara Puente-Marín and
María del Mar Ortega-Villaizan*
Instituto de Biología Molecular y Celular, Universidad Miguel Hernandez, Elche, Spain

*Address all correspondence to: mortega-villaizan@umh.es

References

[1] Khandelwal S, Saxena RK. A role of phosphatidylserine externalization in clearance of erythrocytes exposed to stress but not in eliminating aging populations of erythrocyte in mice. Experimental Gerontology. 2008;**43**(8): 764-770

[2] Moras M, Lefevre SD, Ostuni MA. From erythroblasts to mature red blood cells: Organelle clearance in mammals. Frontiers in Physiology. 2017;**8**:1076

[3] Morera D et al. RNA-Seq reveals an integrated immune response in nucleated erythrocytes. PLoS One. 2011; **6**(10):e26998

[4] Grasso P, Gangolli S, Gaunt I. Essentials of Pathology for Toxicologists. Florida, USA: CRC Press Inc; 2002

[5] Alberts B et al. Molecular Biology of the Cell. Fourth ed. Garland Science: New York and London; 2002

[6] Morera D, Mackenzie SA. Is there a direct role for erythrocytes in the immune response? Veterinary Research. 2011;**42**(1):89

[7] Janeway CA Jr. Approaching the asymptote? Evolution and revolution in immunology. Cold Spring Harbor Symposia on Quantitative Biology. 1989; **54**(Pt 1):1-13

[8] Janeway CA, Medzhitov R. Innate immune recognition. Annual Review of Immunology. 2002;**20**(1):197-216

[9] Creagh EM, O'Neill LA. TLRs, NLRs and RLRs: A trinity of pathogen sensors that co-operate in innate immunity. Trends in Immunology. 2006;**27**(8): 352-357

[10] St Paul M et al. Chicken erythrocytes respond to toll-like receptor ligands by up-regulating cytokine transcripts. Research in Veterinary Science. 2013;**95**(1):87-91

[11] Rodriguez MF et al. Characterization of toll-like receptor 3 gene in rainbow trout (*Oncorhynchus mykiss*). Immunogenetics. 2005;**57**(7): 510-519

[12] Wessel O et al. Piscine orthoreovirus (PRV) replicates in Atlantic salmon (*Salmo salar L.*) erythrocytes ex vivo. Veterinary Research. 2015;**46**:26

[13] Shen Y et al. Fish red blood cells express immune genes and responses. Aquaculture and Fisheries. 2018;**3**(1): 14-21

[14] Iqbal M, Philbin VJ, Smith AL. Expression patterns of chicken toll-like receptor mRNA in tissues, immune cell subsets and cell lines. Veterinary Immunology and Immunopathology. 2005;**104**(1–2):117-127

[15] Cormier F. Avian pluripotent haemopoietic progenitor cells: Detection and enrichment from the para-aortic region of the early embryo. Journal of Cell Science. 1993;**105**(Pt 3):661-666

[16] Nombela I, Ortega-Villaizan MDM. Nucleated red blood cells: Immune cell mediators of the antiviral response. PLoS Pathogens. 2018;**14**(4):e1006910

[17] Robertsen B. The interferon system of teleost fish. Fish & Shellfish Immunology. 2006;**20**(2):172-191

[18] Zou J, Bird S, Secombes C. Antiviral sensing in teleost fish. Current Pharmaceutical Design. 2010;**16**(38): 4185-4193

[19] Schultz U, Kaspers B, Staeheli P. The interferon system of non-mammalian vertebrates. Developmental

and Comparative Immunology. 2004; **28**(5):499-508

[20] Schneider WM, Chevillotte MD, Rice CM. Interferon-stimulated genes: A complex web of host defenses. Annual Review of Immunology. 2014;**32**: 513-545

[21] Liang SL, Quirk D, Zhou A. RNase L: Its biological roles and regulation. IUBMB Life. 2006;**58**(9):508-514

[22] Workenhe ST et al. Infectious salmon anaemia virus replication and induction of alpha interferon in Atlantic salmon erythrocytes. Virology Journal. 2008;**5**:36

[23] Dahle MK et al. Transcriptome analyses of Atlantic salmon (*Salmo salar L.*) erythrocytes infected with piscine orthoreovirus (PRV). Fish & Shellfish Immunology. 2015;**45**(2):780-790

[24] Haatveit HM et al. Viral protein kinetics of piscine orthoreovirus infection in atlantic Salmon blood cells. Viruses. 2017;**9**(3):49

[25] Nombela I et al. Infectious pancreatic necrosis virus triggers antiviral immune response in rainbow trout red blood cells, despite not being infective. F1000Research. 2017;**6**:1968

[26] Nombela I et al. Identification of diverse defense mechanisms in rainbow trout red blood cells in response to halted replication of VHS virus. F1000Research. 2017;**6**:1958

[27] Medzhitov R. Toll-like receptors and innate immunity. Nature Reviews. Immunology. 2001;**1**(2):135-145

[28] Kaiser MG et al. Cytokine expression in chicken peripheral blood mononuclear cells after in vitro exposure to Salmonella enterica serovar Enteritidis. Poultry Science. 2006; **85**(11):1907-1911

[29] Bystry RS et al. B cells and professional APCs recruit regulatory T cells via CCL4. Nature Immunology. 2001;**2**(12):1126-1132

[30] Kogut MH. Dynamics of a protective avian inflammatory response: The role of an IL-8-like cytokine in the recruitment of heterophils to the site of organ invasion by Salmonella enteritidis. Comparative Immunology, Microbiology and Infectious Diseases. 2002;**25**(3):159-172

[31] Cui L et al. Immunoregulatory function of neonatal nucleated red blood cells in humans. Immunobiology. 2016; **221**(8):853-861

[32] Seledtsova GV et al. A role for interferon-gamma and transforming growth factor-beta in erythroid cell-mediated regulation of nitric oxide production in macrophages. Immunology. 1997;**91**(1):109-113

[33] Passantino L et al. Antigenically activated avian erythrocytes release cytokine-like factors: A conserved phylogenetic function discovered in fish. Immunopharmacology and Immunotoxicology. 2007;**29**(1):141-152

[34] Chico V et al. Shape-shifted red blood cells: A novel red blood cell stage? Cell. 2018;**7**(4):E31

[35] Yi Y et al. High-throughput identification of antimicrobial peptides from amphibious mudskippers. Marine Drugs. 2017;**15**(11):E364

[36] Smith VJ, Desbois AP, Dyrynda EA. Conventional and unconventional antimicrobials from fish, marine invertebrates and micro-algae. Marine Drugs. 2010;**8**(4):1213-1262

[37] Peschel A, Sahl HG. The co-evolution of host cationic antimicrobial peptides and microbial resistance. Nature Reviews. Microbiology. 2006; **4**(7):529-536

[38] Casadei E et al. Characterization of three novel beta-defensin antimicrobial peptides in rainbow trout (*Oncorhynchus mykiss*). Molecular Immunology. 2009; **46**(16):3358-3366

[39] Ellis AE. Innate host defense mechanisms of fish against viruses and bacteria. Developmental and Comparative Immunology. 2001;**25** (8–9):827-839

[40] Pereiro P et al. Nucleated teleost erythrocytes play an Nk-Lysin- and autophagy-dependent role in antiviral immunity. Frontiers in Immunology. 2017;**8**:1458

[41] Andersson M et al. NK-lysin, a novel effector peptide of cytotoxic T and NK cells. Structure and cDNA cloning of the porcine form, induction by interleukin 2, antibacterial and antitumour activity. The EMBO Journal. 1995;**14**(8): 1615-1625

[42] Pena SV, Krensky AM. Granulysin, a new human cytolytic granule-associated protein with possible involvement in cell-mediated cytotoxicity. Seminars in Immunology. 1997;**9**(2):117-125

[43] Clayberger C et al. 15 kDa granulysin causes differentiation of monocytes to dendritic cells but lacks cytotoxic activity. Journal of Immunology. 2012;**188**(12):6119-6126

[44] Krause A et al. LEAP-1, a novel highly disulfide-bonded human peptide, exhibits antimicrobial activity. FEBS Letters. 2000;**480** (2–3):147-150

[45] Wang KJ et al. Cloning and expression of a hepcidin gene from a marine fish (*Pseudosciaena crocea*) and the antimicrobial activity of its synthetic peptide. Peptides. 2009;**30**(4):638-646

[46] Douglas SE et al. Identification and expression analysis of hepcidin-like antimicrobial peptides in bony fish. Developmental and Comparative Immunology. 2003;**27**(6–7):589-601

[47] Hirono I et al. Two different types of hepcidins from the Japanese flounder *Paralichthys olivaceus*. The FEBS Journal. 2005;**272**(20):5257-5264

[48] Gui L et al. Two hepcidins from spotted scat (*Scatophagus argus*) possess antibacterial and antiviral functions in vitro. Fish & Shellfish Immunology. 2016;**50**:191-199

[49] Kawasaki H, Iwamuro S. Potential roles of histones in host defense as antimicrobial agents. Infectious Disorders Drug Targets. 2008;**8**(3): 195-205

[50] Rose-Martel M, Hincke MT. Antimicrobial histones from chicken erythrocytes bind bacterial cell wall lipopolysaccharides and lipoteichoic acids. International Journal of Antimicrobial Agents. 2014;**44**(5): 470-472

[51] Rose-Martel M et al. Histones from avian erythrocytes exhibit antibiofilm activity against methicillin-sensitive and methicillin-resistant *Staphylococcus aureus*. Scientific Reports. 2017;**7**:45980

[52] Jodoin J, Hincke MT. Histone H5 is a potent antimicrobial agent and a template for novel antimicrobial peptides. Scientific Reports. 2018;**8**(1): 2411

[53] Jiang N et al. Respiratory protein-generated reactive oxygen species as an antimicrobial strategy. Nature Immunology. 2007;**8**(10):1114-1122

[54] Minasyan HA. Erythrocyte and leukocyte: Two partners in bacteria killing. International Reviews of Immunology. 2014;**33**(6):490-497

[55] Thielen AJF, Zeerleder S, Wouters D. Consequences of dysregulated

complement regulators on red blood cells. Blood Reviews. 2018;**32**:280-288

[56] Schraml B, Baker MA, Reilly BD. A complement receptor for opsonized immune complexes on erythrocytes from *Oncorhynchus mykiss* but not *Ictalarus punctatus*. Molecular Immunology. 2006;**43**(10):1595-1603

[57] Schifferli JA, Ng YC, Peters DK. The role of complement and its receptor in the elimination of immune complexes. The New England Journal of Medicine. 1986;**315**(8):488-495

[58] Krych-Goldberg M, Atkinson JP. Structure-function relationships of complement receptor typ. 1. Immunological Reviews. 2001;**180**: 112-122

[59] Carlisle RC et al. Human erythrocytes bind and inactivate typ. 5 adenovirus by presenting Coxsackie virus-adenovirus receptor and complement receptor 1. Blood. 2009; **113**(9):1909-1918

[60] Espenes A et al. Immune-complex trapping in the splenic ellipsoids of rainbow trout (*Oncorhynchus mykiss*). Cell and Tissue Research. 1995;**282**(1): 41-48

[61] Akintude ME, Heuer L, Van de Water J. Immune abnormalities and autism spectrum disorders. Editors: Joseph D. Buxbaum, Patrick R. Hof. Academic Press. In: The Neuroscience of Autism Spectrum Disorders. 2013. pp. 233-248. ISBN 9780123919243

[62] Janeway CA et al. Immunobiology. 6th ed. Garland Science; 2005. ISBN 0443073104

[63] Sarder MR et al. The MHC class I linkage group is a major determinant in the in vivo rejection of allogeneic erythrocytes in rainbow trout (*Oncorhynchus mykiss*). Immunogenetics. 2003;**55**(5):315-324

[64] Nedelkovska H et al. Effective RNAi-mediated beta2-microglobulin loss of function by transgenesis in *Xenopus laevis*. Biology Open. 2013;**2**(3): 335-342

[65] Delany ME et al. Cellular expression of MHC glycoproteins on erythrocytes from normal and aneuploid chickens. Developmental and Comparative Immunology. 1987;**11**(3):613-625

[66] Villadangos JA, Schnorrer P, Wilson NS. Control of MHC class II antigen presentation in dendritic cells: A balance between creative and destructive forces. Immunological Reviews. 2005;**207**: 191-205

[67] Puente-Marin S et al. In silico functional networks identified in fish nucleated red blood cells by means of transcriptomic and proteomic profiling. Genes (Basel). 2018;**9**(4):E202

[68] Fonseca AM et al. Red blood cells promote survival and cell cycle progression of human peripheral blood T cells independently of CD58/LFA-3 and heme compounds. Cellular Immunology. 2003;**224**(1):17-28

[69] Shau H, Gupta RK, Golub SH. Identification of a natural killer enhancing factor (NKEF) from human erythroid cells. Cellular Immunology. 1993;**147**(1):1-11

[70] Passantino L et al. Fish immunology. I. Binding and engulfment of *Candida albicans* by erythrocytes of rainbow trout (*Salmo gairdneri* Richardson). Immunopharmacology and Immunotoxicology. 2002;**24**(4): 665-678

[71] Humphrey MB, Lanier LL, Nakamura MC. Role of ITAM-containing adapter proteins and their receptors in the immune system and bone. Immunological Reviews. 2005; **208**:50-65

[72] Ohashi K et al. A molecule in teleost fish, related with human MHC-encoded G6F, has a cytoplasmic tail with ITAM and marks the surface of thrombocytes and in some fishes also of erythrocytes. Immunogenetics. 2010;**62**(8):543-559

[73] Gatto D et al. Guidance of B cells by the orphan G protein-coupled receptor EBI2 shapes humoral immune responses. Immunity. 2009;**31**(2): 259-269

[74] Gotting M, Nikinmaa MJ. Transcriptomic analysis of young and old erythrocytes of fish. Frontiers in Physiology. 2017;**8**:1046

[75] Xia J, Gill EE, Hancock RE. Network analyst for statistical, visual and network-based meta-analysis of gene expression data. Nature Protocols. 2015; **10**(6):823-844

Chapter 4

Multifunctional Activity of the β-Defensin-2 during Respiratory Infections

Dora Patricia Rosete Olvera and Carlos Cabello Gutiérrez

Abstract

Human β-defensin-2 is a small cationic peptide that is part of the innate and adaptive immunity. It is expressed mainly in the epithelium and has a broad spectrum of antimicrobial activity against bacteria, fungi and viruses. In addition to its antimicrobial activity, it has other biological functions. The alteration of the expression of β-defensin-2 in the respiratory epithelium has been associated with the pathogenesis of several respiratory diseases such as asthma, pulmonary fibrosis, pneumonia, tuberculosis, rhinitis, etc. The acute respiratory infections caused by viruses are the main cause of morbidity and mortality in the world; there are few studies and it is necessary to study this peptide to understand its role in the viral pathogenesis. In addition, it also becomes relevant in its potential to take advantage of its properties in the development of alternative therapies that allow the prevention or treatment of viral respiratory infections.

Keywords: β-defensin-2, pathogenesis, respiratory diseases, viral infections

1. Introduction

Defensins are a family of antimicrobial peptides that are part of the innate and adaptive immune system. They provide protection against too broad spectrum of pathogens, viruses, bacteria and fungi [1]. The defensins are small cationic peptides of 3–4 kb, and its structure is composed of beta sheets, six cysteines joined by disulfide bonds. In humans, it is classified in two groups: α- and β-defensins [2, 3]. The β-defensin-2 (HBD2) is found in the second group and it is a peptide of 41 amino acids; it is expressed mainly in the epithelial cells, mucous and skin [1, 4, 5]. It was isolated in 1997 from skin lesions in patients with psoriasis; later, it was detected in the epithelium of almost entire human body [6–14]. In recent years, HBD2 has been considered as a multifunctional peptide with antimicrobial activity and with immunomodulatory functions [15–17]. On the other hand, the HBD2 is expressed throughout the respiratory epithelium from the mouth to the lungs; it is believed that this defensin has a very important role in the defense against respiratory infections [2]. The alteration of the expression of the HBD2 in the respiratory epithelium has been associated with the pathogenesis of several respiratory diseases such as asthma, pulmonary fibrosis, pneumonia, tuberculosis, rhinitis, etc. [2, 9, 17–20].

The acute respiratory infections caused by viruses are the main cause of morbidity and mortality in the world, and HBD2 has got antiviral activity against some respiratory viruses (influenza, respiratory syncytial virus, rhinovirus) [21–23]. The mechanisms of viral inactivation vary and include not only direct binding of the virus to the peptide but also indirect methods of inactivation via intracellular modulation of the viral replication, modulation of signaling pathways necessary for antiviral effects, and recruitment of immune cells that contribute to antiviral activity [2, 22]. This revision chapter focuses on the structural and general characteristics of HBD2, multifunctional activities and expression in respiratory diseases. We present some studies concerning the effect of respiratory viruses and their relationship with HBD2, mechanisms of action and their relevance as therapeutic agents.

2. General characteristics and classification

Defensins are a family of antimicrobial peptides that form part of the innate and adaptive immune system and constitute the first line of host defense against microorganisms. It has shown the broad antimicrobial activity spectrum against bacteria, fungi and viruses [1, 24].

The defensins are small cationic peptides of 28–42 amino acids, characterized by a β-sheet structure linked by tree disulfide bonds, which are formed by six cysteine residues [2, 25]. Based on the distribution of their cysteines and disulfide bonds, defensins are classified into two groups in humans: α- and β-defensins [1]. α-defensins have 29–35 amino acids and the positions of the cysteines are C1-C6, C2-C4 and C3-C5, while the β-defensins are composed of 38–42 amino acids with the positions of the cysteines of C1-C5, C2-C4 and C3-C6 [26].

The α-defensins are expressed mainly in neutrophils and called human neutrophil peptides with four types (HNP1–4). There are other α-defensins (HD5 and HD6), known as enteric defensins, that are expressed in Paneth cells in the small intestine [27]. The expression of HBD6 has also been confirmed in the female genitourinary system [1, 28].

β-defensins are mainly expressed in epithelial cells throughout the body, including mucous membranes and skin [29–32]. Four types (HBD1–4) have been identified in humans, but several analyses indicate that there may be approximately 31 types, of which HBD5 and 6 are expressed in epididymis with their importance in defense against infections. The other defensins are known only for their antimicrobial activity [33, 34]. The β-defensin-1 is expressed constitutively, while the other three (HBD2–4) are expressed by the effect of proinflammatory cytokines or during the infectious process [1, 28].

3. Molecular structure of β-defensin-2

The HBD2 is a small cationic peptide with a positive net charge (+6). It has 41 amino acid residues; the complete gene is approximately 4 kb. It consists of six cysteines in positions 1–5, 2–4 and 3–6, joined by three disulfide bonds. Its secondary structure consists of an N-terminal region linked to an alpha helix, three β-strands arranged in an antiparallel sheet and a C-terminal region [35–37] (**Figure 1**). Its structure has an amphipathic nature, with hydrophilic and hydrophobic amino acids on the surface of protein; it is stabilized by the disulfide bonds, which protect it from degradation by proteases [38, 39]. The alpha helix is also stabilized by the disulfide bonds (I and V) and by the first beta sheet that has a domain (Gly-X-CysIV), which is responsible for the native structure and the correct folding of the peptide [40, 41]. The N-terminal region binds to the membrane of microorganisms.

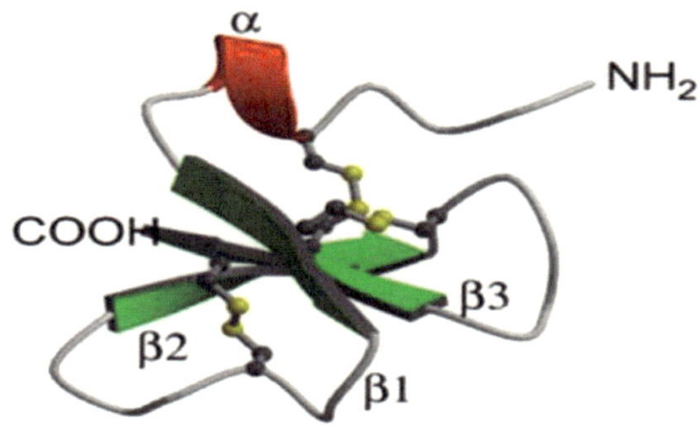

Figure 1.
Secondary structure of HBD-2 that consists of an N-terminal region linked to an alpha helix, three β-strands arranged in an antiparallel sheet and a C-terminal region [41].

The specific conformation of N-terminal region of β-defensins may be important for the biological properties of these proteins. [37].

The C-terminal region consists mainly of cationic amino acids (lysine and arginine) that are distributed asymmetrically with their positive charges and are important in antimicrobial activity [3, 38, 40].

4. Genetic structure of β-defensin-2

The gene codify for HBD2 is located on chromosome 8p23. The gene is approximately 4 kb and composed of a 5'and 3' non-translatable region, two exons separated by an intron. The first exon has 81 bp and codes for the signal peptide and the second exon has 238 bp and codes for a short anion segment called propeptide and the mature peptide [3, 25, 42]. The 5′ region of HBD2 has specific sites that bind to the transcription factor kB (NF-kB). In addition, there are sites that bind to other transcription factors such as C/EBP, and NF-IL-6, which are important for their expression [42–44].

The HBD2 have a polymorphic nature, and the number of copies of the gene varies in each individual [45]. It has been reported that there are 2–12 copies per diploid genome, and the number of copies is related to the level of expression. It has been suggested that these variations may have consequences on the function of immune system. Some infectious and inflammatory diseases are related to the number of copies of the HBD2 gene [44, 46] (**Figure 2**).

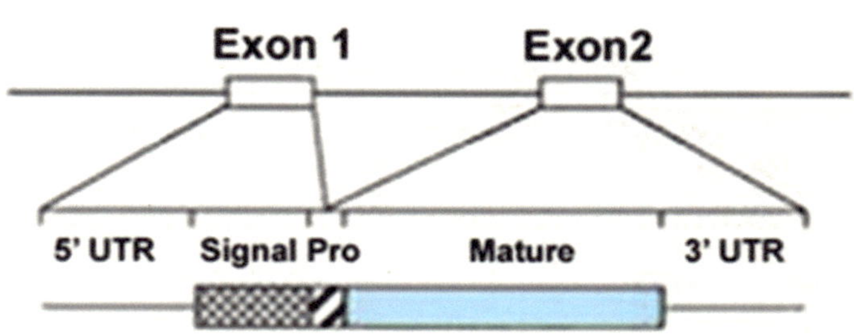

Figure 2.
Genetic structure of HBD2. It encompasses untranslated 5 'and 3' regions and two exons separated by an intron. The first exon codes for the signal peptide and the second exon codes for the propeptide and the mature peptide [3].

5. Expression and regulation of β-defensin-2

HBD2 is expressed mainly in all the epithelia of human body (respiratory, digestive, urogenital, conjunctive epithelium), mucous, peripheral blood and skin. In the respiratory system, HBD2 is expressed in mucous from the mouth to the epithelium of the lungs and is induced by bacteria, fungi and virus infections and by proinflammatory stimuli such as interleukin 1α (IL-1α), interleukin 1β (IL-1β), tumor necrosis factor alpha (TNF-α), interferon gamma (IFN-γ) and interleukin IL-6 (IL-6) [29, 47–51]. Recently, a study showed that the cytokines IL-17 and IL-22 are produced by Th17 cells, which are reportedly known to regulate the expression of HBD2 on mucosal surfaces [32]. HBD2 is produced as a functionally inactive peptide (prepro-defensin), and to achieve its biological activity, it must go through a post-translational modification process and form a mature peptide. Prepro-defensin is composed of a highly hydrophobic pre-peptide signal, a propeptide and the mature peptide. The prepropeptide is cut by proteases in the Golgi apparatus, and once removed, the mature peptide with antimicrobial activity is secreted on the surface of the epithelial cells [3, 52].

The regulation of the expression of the HBD2 in the respiratory epithelium involves multiple signaling pathways; most of these have been studied with bacterial infections. The bacterial proteins induce the expression of HBD2 in the respiratory epithelium through transcription factors (NF-kB) [53], the myeloid ELF-1-like factor (MEF) [54], the nuclear factor interleukin 6 (NF-IL6) [55] or the activated protein 1–3 (AP1–3) [56]. Signaling pathways involve mitogen-activated protein kinase (MAPKs) [49, 57, 58], phosphatidylinositol-3-kinase (PI3K) and protein kinase C (PKC) [59].

Another form to induce HBD2 expression is through cellular receptors, the respiratory epithelium expresses various receptors on its surface. Toll-like receptors (TLRs) 1–6 are expressed on the epithelial surface, and in the intracellular vesicles, the TLR3 and TLR7–9 are expressed in the endosomes or endoplasmic reticulum. These receptors recognize pathogens and have a cytoplasmic domain that is homologous to the IL-1 receptor and is responsible for initiating intracellular signaling pathways. This signaling cascade includes the activation of NF-kB. This transcription factor promotes the gene expression that contributes to the cytokines, chemokines, adhesion molecules, co-stimulatory molecules release as well as the expression of HBD2 [60].

In a study with lung epithelial cells infected with *L. pneumophila*, it was observed that the infection induces the release of HBD2, and its expression is mediated by the receptors TLR2 and TLR5 and activation of MAPKs (p38, JNK) and transcription factors NF-kB and AP-1 [50, 57, 58, 61].

Another way to regulate the expression of HBD2 is through the interaction with receptors; its chemotactic property was initially discovered in different types of cells such as monocytes, T cells and immature dendritic cells. The activity is carried through the CCR6 receptor binding [32].

Other receptors involved in the regulation of the HBD2 expression are the receptors for vitamin D and protease-coupled receptors (PARs) [62–65].

Nowadays, HBD2 is considered a multifunctional molecule; the ability to bind to several ligands suggests that there may be more receptors and signaling pathways still to be discovered and that may have important biological activities in the immune system.

6. Mechanisms of action of β-defensin-2

Several mechanisms of action have been proposed for defensins; however, the main mechanism of action of the HBD2 is to eliminate microorganisms

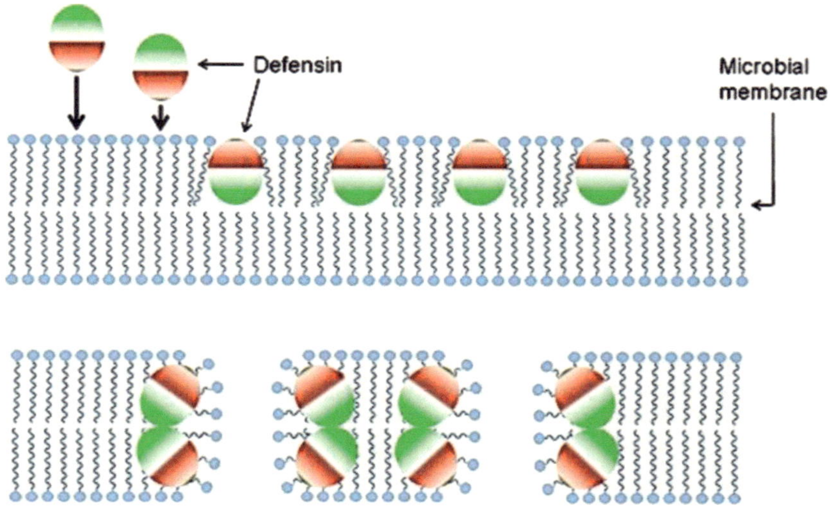

Figure 3.
Mechanisms of action of HBD2. The defensin with its positive charge is attached by electrostatic attraction to the membrane of the pathogen forming pores [3].

directly through the interaction with the microorganism membrane. The first step is given by the electrostatic attraction between the cationic defensin with positive charge and the microorganism's membrane components with negative charges [37].

Components of the bacteria membrane have been identified as targets for the HBD2. Lipopolysaccharides are targets for Gram-negative bacteria, teichoic acid for Gram-positive bacteria and phospholipids for both bacteria. In Gram-negative bacteria, the peptides are inserted into the membrane by hydrophobic interactions. It is thought that it possibly involves a folding of the peptide within the structure of the membrane [38, 66, 67]. After the electrostatic interaction of the peptide with the membrane and the displacement of the lipids, the defensin is added to the surface of membrane. There are several modes of action that have been proposed to describe how defensins are oriented to form pores and how the structure of the membrane is altered, becomes permeable, such as cell lysis and finally results in the death of the microorganism (**Figure 3**) [3, 37, 68].

The high content of negatively charged amino acids in the membranes of bacteria is the main factor that makes them more susceptible to being targeted by defensins. The membrane of the eukaryotic cells predominates lipids with neutral charge without net charge, they have a high level of cholesterol, and bacteria do not contain cholesterol in their membranes. Cholesterol causes the membrane to condense and prevents the peptide from penetrating; this also has an asymmetric distribution of phospholipids contributing to the resistance against defensing. These mechanisms explain why these peptides are not toxic in eukaryotic cells [69, 70].

7. Multifunctional activities of β-defensin-2

HBD2 was isolated and characterized by its antimicrobial activity. Currently, several studies have described different biological activities of HBD2, and it is considered as a multifunctional protein. Some of the account on its biological activities is given below.

7.1 Antimicrobial activities

HBD2 has a broad spectrum of activity against a wide variety of bacteria, fungi and viruses. The mechanism of action of this defensin begins with the interaction of the negative charges of the pathogen membrane, the formation of pores and finally the lysis of the microorganism. The variability of the composition of the membranes of the different pathogens explains in part the different antimicrobial effects [2, 22].

7.2 Innate and adaptive immunity

HBD2 is important in innate immunity and constitutes the first line of host defense against infections by microorganisms. Its role in adaptive immunity is attributed mainly to its chemotactic activity in immature dendritic cells and memory T lymphocytes through the CCR6 receptor [26].

Several mechanisms have been proposed for HBD2 that contributes to the adaptive immunity: (a) Increase in the recruitment of immature dendritic cells. Immature dendritic cells are recruited from circulating blood or tissue near the site of inflammation by chemoattractants that interact with their corresponding receptors (CCR1, CCR5, CCR6). (b) Formation of defensin-antigen complexes. HBD2 forms defensin-antigen complexes facilitating the presentation to dendritic cells. (c) Maturation of dendritic cells. HBD2 induced the maturation of dendritic cells for direct production of IL-2 or indirect production of TNF and IL-1 by monocytes and macrophages. (d) Recruitment of memory T cells. It facilitates the recruitment of memory T cells that are the effector cells of adaptive immunity [15, 26].

HBD2 contributes to unite the innate and adaptive immune response, and this property has been applied for the development of vaccine adjuvants, since it promotes adaptive immunity when it is administered together with antigens [15, 26].

7.3 Inflammation

Inflammation is a protective reaction by the host to eliminate injurious stimuli (microorganism, damage cell or irritants). Some viral infections cause severe inflammation, and the tissue can be damaged and then it must be repaired. The mechanisms include the production of anti-inflammatory cytokines, lipid mediators, glucocorticoids, immune cell apoptosis, etc. [3].

HBD2 plays a critical role in regulating inflammation processes in the respiratory system and modulates the production of inflammatory cytokines and chemokines. An increase in local expression has been observed; but in severe cases, the HBD2 can be detected systemically [71].

HBD-2 can promote histamine release and prostaglandin D2 production in mast cells, suggesting a role in allergic reactions [1, 26, 72].

7.4 Anti-inflammatory activity

HBD2 and the complement system are two important innate immune mechanisms against a broad range of microorganisms. The complement is composed of more than 30 proteins found in the human serum, and it is activated by three different pathways (classical, alternative and lectin) [73, 74]. It has been described that HBD2 binds to C1q (first component of the complement system) and inhibits the classical complement pathway. HBD2 have a dual protective role not only as an antimicrobial agent but also to provide protection against uncontrolled activation of complement system [73, 75, 76].

7.5 Immunomodulatory properties

Recently, the study of the HBD2 has focused on the modulation of the immune response. It has been suggested that multiple mechanisms of action may be involved from direct binding to the membrane of the microorganism to the union with different types of cellular receptors that can induce transduction signals, gene transcription and various signaling pathways [77]. This mechanism paves the way for the development of new therapies for infectious respiratory diseases.

7.5.1 Moxifloxacin/HBD2

In a study with epithelial lung cells (A549) stimulated with LPS, it was demonstrated that the association of moxifloxacin/HBD2 has an anti-inflammatory effect. Moxifloxacin is a fluoroquinolone against Gram-positive and Gram-negative bacteria, which may have affected the immune system. The treatment induced a reduction of proinflammatory cytokines (IL-1 and IL-6). These data support the hypothesis of its immunomodulatory capacity of HBD2 to neutralize the components of bacteria that induce the activation of cytokines [78].

7.5.2 Vitamin D (VitD)

VitD plays an important role for the calcium homeostasis in the bones. Currently, the interest has focused on the modulation of the immune response in fighting viral respiratory infections. Some studies show that patients with deficiencies in VitD are at higher risk of suffering respiratory infections in the upper respiratory tract [79]. One study showed the association of polymorphisms in the VitD receptor and severe bronchiolitis in patients infected by the respiratory syncytial virus [80].

The immunomodulatory effect has been of great importance in some viral infections; several types of cells including epithelial cells treated with VitD induce the expression of the receptor and the production of antimicrobial peptides such as the HBD2. In the patients infected with HIV, the high levels of VitD and its receptor increase the amount of IL-10 and HBD2, which are associated with a natural resistance to HIV infection [62].

The VitD receptor is expressed in several types of cells (monocytes, B cells, T cells and NK), is an endogenous immunomodulator and induces the transcription of the HBD2. This work shows that the expression of HBD2 is important to render tolerance to viral infections [62, 64].

7.5.3 PARs (receptors coupled to proteases)

It is a family of receptors coupled to the G-protein, which is formed by seven transmembrane domains with an amino-terminal extracellular domain and a C-terminal domain. PARs are activated by proteolytic cleavage in the N-terminal domain by serine proteases. N-terminal serves as a ligand to carry out intracellular signaling. They are expressed in epithelial, endothelial and immune cells such as leukocytes, mast cells, eosinophils, neutrophils and mastoid cells. Four types of receptors have been described (PAR-1–4). PAR-1, 3 and 4 are activated mainly by thrombin and are involved in the aggregation of platelets. PAR-2 is activated by trypsin, tryptase from mastoid cells, protease 3 from neutrophils and tissue factor, factor VIIa and Xa [81]. Recently, PARs have been implicated in the regulation of the expression of antimicrobial peptides found in epithelial cells such as defensins [65, 82]. The researchers identified the expression of the HBD2 in human gingiva by *P. gingivalis* infection. Further, proteases of the bacteria induced the expression of the defensin through PAR2. The authors suggest that this signaling pathway can lead to the development of preventive therapies in mucosal infections [65].

7.5.4 Triptolide

This is an immunosuppressive and anti-inflammatory agent that was extracted from an herb of Chinese origin (*Tripterygium wilfordii*). It decreases the expression of the NF-kB and genes related to inflammatory processes. This review chapter shows that this agent suppresses the expression of HBD2 induced by IL-1β in A549 cells and the suppression is associated with the inhibition of NF-kB [83].

7.5.5 Neutrophilic elastase

It is a serine protease that is expressed in neutrophils and stored in their granules. It has been reported that neutrophilic elastase in the bronchial epithelium has a direct effect against bacteria; in addition, it can regulate the increased expression of the HBD2 [84].

7.5.6 Dexamethasone

It is a synthetic glucocorticoid that is used in the treatment of respiratory, allergic or autoimmune diseases. Its effect is to decrease the expression of proinflammatory cytokine genes through NF-kB. The clinical use of glucocorticoids can increase the susceptibility to infections by decreasing the expression of antimicrobial peptides such as the HBD2. In this study, they investigated the molecular mechanism by which dexamethasone modulated HBD2 expression in response to IL-1b in A549 cells and, the role of MAPKs, MKP-1, AKT, and NF-kB transcription factor. They demonstrated that dexamethasone suppresses the expression of HBD2 for this signaling pathway [83].

7.5.7 Isoleucine

Isoleucine is an essential amino acid that can induce the expression of the HBD2 in the epithelium. Its expression involves the activation of NF-kB/rel family of trans-activating factors. The authors suggest that isoleucine or analogues may have clinical utility as immunostimulants that could bolster the defense of the respiratory epithelium and mucosae [85].

7.5.8 Hyaluronic acid

When the skin epithelium suffers damage, the hyaluronic acid, which is found in the extracellular matrix, is fragmented and activates keratinocytes which in turn stimulate the HBD2 production. The induction is mediated by toll receptors (TLR2 and TLR4) as well as other signaling pathways such as c-Fos and protein kinase C; thus, the epithelium is protected from infections [86].

7.5.9 Sirtuin1 (SIRT1)

It is a nicotinamide adenine dinucleotide-dependent histone deacetylase, which regulates several processes of the innate and adaptive immune system.

The anti-inflammatory properties of SIRT1 are reportedly known to show [87] that the infection with *S. pneumoniae* in alveolar epithelial cells (A549) induces HBD2 production involving the SIRT1. Furthermore, HBD2 production induced by *S pneumoniae* is mediated by the MAPK activation (p38), and the expression of IL-8 is regulated by the phosphorylation of ERK.

7.6 Wound repair

This process has been described in the epithelium of skin and can be achieved by various means, which includes the modulation of cytokines production, cell proliferation and migration and in some cases angiogenesis [88, 89]. It has been demonstrated that HBD2 is expressed in normal skin [90], and its expression increases when the skin is damaged or during the chronic infection [91].

Patients with diabetes mellitus suffer from skin ulcers, and the expression of HBD2 does not increase when compared to normal skin. The scarce expression of HBD2 is seen during the chronic disease. The authors supposed that high glucose levels inhibit the expression of HBD2 in human keratinocytes [92].

HBD2 is reportedly seen to elicit intracellular Ca^{+2} mobilization and increased keratinocyte migration and proliferation [93]. Besides, this peptide induced phosphorylation of EGFR, signal transducer and activator of transcription STAT1 and STAT3. These are intracellular signaling molecules involved in keratinocyte migration and proliferation.

7.7 Angiogenesis

It is a process by which endothelial cells proliferate and migrate towards the angiogenic stimulus to form new blood vessels. This process is part of the repair of damaged tissues and severe inflammatory processes. The present paper demonstrates that HBD2 stimulates the migration, proliferation and formation of capillary tubes of endothelial cells [94].

7.8 Cytokines and chemokines

Peripheral blood mononuclear cells when stimulated by the HBD2 induce a strong cytokine response. The cytokines that were detected in the highest concentration were interleukin 6 (IL-6), interleukin 8 (IL-8) and interleukin 10 (IL10). It was also found that monocyte chemotactic protein 1 (MCP-1) induces a strong response and also induces RANTES, IL-1β, ENA-78 and GRO, so that the induction patterns of cytokines/chemokines can be crucial in the development and amplification of the immune response against pathogenic microorganisms [95].

7.9 Hypertension

It has been proven that HBD2 can regulate blood pressure and provide a new mechanism for the treatment of hypertension [96].

8. Respiratory diseases associated with the expression of β-defensin-2

The respiratory epithelium is the largest surface of the human body in contact with external medium, and it exposed to a large number of pathogens.

The respiratory epithelium counts upon many defense effectors and one of them is the production of defensins. They act as a first line of host defense against invading microorganism. The cells of respiratory epithelium produce four types of defensins (HBD1–4). HBD1 is expressed constitutively and HBD2–4 are expressed during infectious or inflammatory processes. HBD2 is the most expressed in all respiratory epithelium from the oral cavity, pharynx, larynx, trachea, serous cells and submucosal glands to the lung [1, 29, 97]. Several authors have reported expression of the HBD2 in these tissues and also detected the protein in healthy and diseased people in different secretions of the body such as bronchoalveolar fluid, saliva, blood, plasma, milk, sputum, nasal secretions, etc. [32, 98–102].

Several studies have suggested that there is a relationship between HBD2 and the pathogenesis of several respiratory diseases. The increase or decrease of its expression can result in the protection or amplification of the disease.

8.1 Lung cancer

This type of disease has a high mortality rate and the treatments are very expensive. It is difficult to detect early stages of the disease or if the tumor is benign or malignant, especially in the preliminary condition. The higher concentrations of HBD2 in the serum of patients did not show any relation with the histopathological classification [103].

8.2 Pneumonia

It is a disease of the lower respiratory system that mainly affects young children and older adults and has a high mortality rate and a great social and economic impact due to long periods of hospitalization and resistance to antibiotics. The alteration of the immune function of the mucosa of the respiratory system in these age groups constitutes a risk factor for contracting pneumonia. Bacterial infections are frequent, such infections lead to a serious deterioration of lung function, and are usually associated with persistent colonization by bacteria such as *Pseudomonas aeruginosa, Haemophilus influenzae, Streptococcus pneumonia* and *Legionella pneumophila.* Patients with acute pneumonia caused by bacterial infections have shown that the HBD2 is expressed in lung tissue and the concentration of the protein increases in blood and alveolar fluid [98, 101]. When the HBD2 levels in plasma are below 12.5 mg/ml, the patients with pneumonia have a high possibility of needing mechanical ventilation and development of new complications or death [104].

In an in vitro model, *L. pneumophila* induces the release of hBD-2 in A549 cells in a manner dependent on TLR2 and TLR5. The activation of p38 MAPK and JNK, as well as NF-B and AP-1, is involved in the production of hBD-2 induced by *L. pneumophila*. Therefore, regulation of the release of hBD-2 by *L. pneumophila* in A549 cells appears to be determined by multiple signaling molecules and may contribute to host defense in Legionnaires disease. [57].

8.3 Cystic fibrosis

Cystic fibrosis is a chronic lung disease with high morbidity and mortality rates. It is caused by a recessive mutation in the transmembrane conductance regulator gene (CFTR), which is located on chromosome 7 on the apical surface of epithelial cells [19, 24, 105]. This mutation causes abnormal transport of chlorine ions, which induce an increase in the salinity of the alveolar fluid. The high salt concentration abrogates the antimicrobial activity of HBD2; this might explain the recurrent bacterial infections in the lungs of these patients [32, 105].

Bacterial infections in patients with cystic fibrosis are very common; in the acute phase, the patients are infected mainly with *Haemophilus influenzae* and *Staphylococcus aureus*. While in the chronic phase, the infection is always caused by *Pseudomonas aeruginosa*, a Gram-negative bacterium, opportunistic and resistant to antibiotics [32].

The decrease in the expression and degradation of HBD2 plays an important role in the pathogenesis of pulmonary infection for *P. aeruginosa* in patients with cystic fibrosis [105]. They explain that in the chronic phase of infection, the phenotype of the bacteria changes and it loses the flagella. The flagella are composed of flagellin, which is a virulence factor that promotes mobility and adhesion. The flagellum is the ligand that triggers the signaling pathway for the expression of HBD2. When losing the flagella, the bacterium does not recognize the receptor (TLR5) of the epithelium and transcription of the gene is not executed through NF-kB. The bacterium causes damage to the epithelium of the lung producing a severe inflammatory process, with production of IL-8. IL-8 causes the accumulation of neutrophils; later, they enter apoptosis and phagocytosed by macrophages. Many macrophages accumulate in the lung and secrete cathepsin, a cysteine protease that remodels the extracellular matrix found in large quantities in bronchoalveolar lavage. This enzyme degrades the disulfide bonds of the defensins by inactivating them, thus losing their antimicrobial activity [9].

The patients with cystic fibrosis and polyps showed high levels of HBD2 and TLR2 expression with an increase in IL-8 [106]. In nasal epithelium of patients with CF, HBD2 is not upregulated in response to inflammatory stimuli. The higher levels of inflammatory markers were seen but without any correlation with the expression of HBD2. They explain that the epithelium of patients with cystic fibrosis is chronically exposed to inflammatory stimuli and lost the capacity to upregulate defensin synthesis. The inflammatory stimuli may not be the sole inducers of defense expression [107].

8.4 Chronic obstructive pulmonary disease (COPD)

COPD is an inflammatory disease of the respiratory tract that is characterized by recurrent infections, severe inflammation and is associated with a reduction of airflow and a decrease in lung function [108]. The main environmental risk factor is smoking; some authors suggest that tobacco smoke inhibits the activation of the host's innate immune system. The *in vitro* studies with respiratory epithelium exposed to tobacco smoke are reported to inhibit the expression of HBD2 when infected with bacterium [109]. COPD patients who smoke have lowered basal hBD-2 expression in the epithelial cells of the central airways, which correlates with the amount of cigarette pack years. The decreased HBD2 expression is associated with current or former smoking, which makes the population more susceptible towards infections by microorganisms [108, 110].

Moreover, genetic factors can contribute to the progression of the disease. The variation in the number of copies of HBD2 gene in epithelial cells is associated with the pathogenesis of the disease [110]. Moreover, genetic factors can contribute to the progression of the disease. The variation in the number of copies of HBD2 gene in epithelial cells is associated with the pathogenesis of COPD. In this study showed a significantly higher proportion of the patients with severe COPD had high diploid β-defensin copy numbers (five or more) compared with the control sample.

In another study, the expression of HBD2 in peripheral lung tissue in patients with COPD is elevated and associated with the habit of smoking and with the high levels of IL-8 as well as severity of the disease [111].

8.5 Allergic rhinitis (AR)

AR is an inflammatory disorder that occurs in the nasal mucosa and triggered by the exposure to allergens (mites, pets, insects, pollen, latex items, tobacco particles, ozone, nitrogen oxide, sulfur dioxide, aspirin, etc.) producing inflammation mediated by IgE. Clinically, it is characterized by symptoms such as rhinorrhea, sneezing, nasal congestion and itching. These symptoms worsen a person's productivity and quality of life and cause sleep disturbances, fatigue or depression. Although it occurs more frequently in young children, adults are affected as well [18].

Studies with tonsil tissue (lymphocytes) and pharyngeal epithelial cells from patients with allergic rhinitis found a reduction in the expression of HBD2. When cells are exposed to Th2 cytokines (IL-4, IL-5 and IL-13) and histamine *in vitro*, they also cause a decrease in the expression of HBD2. Therefore, patients with allergic rhinitis are more susceptible to respiratory infections and severe exacerbations [112–114].

8.6 Rhinosinusitis

Rhinosinusitis is characterized by the presence of at least two respiratory symptoms, nasal obstruction and nasal discharge, wherein the presence or absence of nasal polyps is seen. In one study, the sinonasal epithelial cells of patients with rhinosinusitis with nasal polyps showed a decrease in the expression of β-defensin-2 in response to the presence of IL-4 and IL-13 [114–116].

8.7 Otitis media

It is a very common disease mainly affecting the young children under 3 years of age having episode of otitis media. The pathogenesis of the disease is multifactorial, and among the most important factors are viral infections (respiratory syncytial virus, rhinovirus, influenza A, adenovirus) and bacterial infections (Streptococcus pneumoniae, nontypeable *Haemophilus influenzae* (NTHI), and Moraxella catarrhalis). The acute illness resolves quickly but the chronic or recurrent disease can cause hearing loss [39, 117].

The epithelial cells of the middle ear express HBD2, and two signaling pathways have been described. HBD2 expression is induced by pro-inflammatory stimuli such as interleukin 1 alpha (IL-1a), tumor necrosis factor alpha (TNF-a), and lipopolysaccharide (LPS). Their transcriptional activation is mediated through an Src-dependent Raf-MEK1/2-ERK signaling pathway [119]. The other known route is when the bacterium is recognized by the TLR2 of epithelial cells through the MyD88-IRAKI-TRAF6-MKK3/6-p38 MAP kinase signal transduction pathway [117, 118].

8.8 Asthma

It is a common chronic obstructive disease characterized by obstruction, hyperreactivity and inflammation. It affects all age groups throughout the world and has high morbidity and mortality rates [119]. Epidemiological studies indicate that the pathogenesis of asthma is multifactorial. The viral respiratory infections are the main cause of exacerbations or asthma attacks; influenza viruses, parainfluenza, rhinovirus and respiratory syncytial are those that have been identified more frequently [120, 121].

The mechanisms that explain how viruses cause or exacerbate asthma are diverse and some are not yet fully characterized. Recent studies indicate that HBD2 may play an important role in the pathogenesis of asthma. Some mechanisms have been suggested to explain the exacerbations of asthma such as (a) patients with asthma develop a TH2 type response; it induced the production of cytokines (IL-4, IL-5, IL-13) that inhibit the production of HBD2, causing susceptibility to infections [122]. (b) HBD2 induces the activation and degranulation of mastoid cells that release histamine and prostaglandins, substances that increase asthma exacerbations [26].

8.9 Recurrent respiratory papillomatosis

It is a disease in the respiratory tract caused by infection with human papilloma virus. The papilloma virus belongs to the Papovaviridae family. It is a circular double-stranded DNA virus and has no envelope, and its genome is 7200–8000 bp. There are more than 100 serotypes, which due to their oncogenic capacity are divided into high risk and low risk [123].

The disease characterized by abnormal proliferation of epithelial keratinocytes forming a papilloma. It occurs more frequently in the larynx but might spread to the trachea or even lungs. It is common in children 2–4 years of age and in children over 12 years of age and in young adults. The first symptom is progressive dysphonia, with symptoms of variable respiratory obstruction, dyspnea and stridor. Some patients have spontaneous remission and others may have a very rapid growth that may require multiple surgical procedures or cause obstruction resulting in death. Papilloma viruses have a high morbidity rate because of its recurrence, and there are no satisfactory treatments [124, 125].

The serotypes of papilloma that have been found with higher frequency are the serotypes of low risk 6 and 11; nevertheless, a 2% can be infected with other subtypes like the 16 and 18 of high risk, but these are associated with transformation of cells causing carcinoma [123].

The expression of HBD2 in samples of papillomavirus induced lesions in patients with recurrent respiratory papillomatosis, and its association with IL-8 [126] was studied. The lesions showed high levels of HBD2 expression, and the inflammatory process was not significant. Despite the higher expression of HBD2 in the deep-seated tissues, the persistence of the virus leads to the disease progression. They suggest that HBD2 can serve as a signaling molecule to induce the adaptive immune response against viral infection with acceptable inflammatory events.

8.10 Diffuse panbronchiolitis (DP)

DP is a disease with chronic inflammation in the bronchioles of respiratory system. The immune cells are activated, and neutrophils are found in large quantities and activate T lymphocytes. There are often bacterial infections (*P. aeruginosa* and *H influenzae*). The pathogenesis of this disease is not clear; but recently, HBD2 has been implicated. In a study with patients with DP, high levels of HBD2 in bronchoalveolar fluid and plasma were found, suggesting that it could play an important role in the defense against infections. The levels of HBD2 in BAL fluid may be a useful marker of airway inflammation in patients with DPB [127].

8.11 Tuberculosis

Tuberculosis is one of the most frequent infectious diseases that cause more deaths; its incidence is still a global health problem. *Mycobacterium tuberculosis* is the causative agent of tuberculosis, and it can cause a progressive disease or a latent infection. It has been reported that a third part of the population is latently infected and 10% have active disease. There are many difficulties due to highly resistant strains and fewer therapeutic agents [128].

However, HBD2 is suggested to play an important role in the control of the disease by direct inactivation of the bacteria or as an immunostimulant in vaccines. This bacterium mainly infects macrophages and lung epithelial cells. The *in vitro* studies have shown that *M. tuberculosis* induces the expression of HBD2 in human lung epithelial cells (A549) and is associated with the destruction of bacteria [129, 130].

The transfection of monocytes derived from macrophages with the HBD2 gene increases the ability to control the growth of *M tuberculosis* when compared with non-transfected cells [131]. Children infected with *M. tuberculosis* present high concentrations of HBD2 in bronchoalveolar lavage suggesting its involvement in the pathogenesis of disease.

Results are favorable in animal model studies in mice, mice were vaccinated with DNA vaccines (gene encoding β-defensin-2 and antigens of *M tuberculoisis*) and months later were challenged with *M tuberculoisis* strains. The level of protection was evaluated by survival, and tissue damage. DNA vaccines showed protection with significant higher survival and less tissue damage in the mice [132]. When a person is infected with *M. tuberculosis*, the microenvironment is reduced in oxygen; this triggers the expression of the vitamin D receptor and HBD2 inhibits the growth bacteria. The lack of local oxygen benefits the macrophage for its elimination.

Other signaling pathways that have been discovered are in monocytes through the CD40L and IFN receptors that converge in the activation of vitamin D. HBD2 is expressed and acts against the bacterium *M. tuberculosis* [134].

8.12 Sepsis

The infectious diseases can cause severe sepsis and the patient's immune system to suffer drastic changes. This study investigated the concentration and the expression of HBD2 in peripheral whole blood cells from patients with severe sepsis. They detected that the peripheral blood cells expressed a decrease in the expression of HBD2. The patient serum showed higher concentrations of HBD2. The patients with severe sepsis have severe inflammatory processes and the proinflammatory cytokines are at high concentrations (IL-1 and TNF); these cytokines also induce the expression of HBD2. It is suggested that these cytokines may be involved in the overproduction of HBD2 in the blood of patients with sepsis. The decreased HBD2 induced in peripheral blood cells was not associated with decreased plasma levels, suggesting that peripheral blood cells do not represent the exclusive source of released protein [135].

9. Antiviral activity of β-defensin-2 in respiratory infections

The HBD2 was initially studied as an antibacterial peptide, and its antiviral activity has been recently demonstrated. The notion was that it only acted in enveloped viruses, but other studies have proven that they also act against naked viruses and any type of genome DNA, RNA and retroviruses. The mechanisms of antiviral inactivation have been classified as direct and indirect. The direct ones occur when HBD2 binds to the viral membrane by electrostatic attraction, causing pore formation and lysis of microorganism. The indirect mechanism occurs when it inactivates an intracellular pathway of the virus replication cycle or when there is recruitment of immune cells that contribute to their antiviral activity [2].

Acute respiratory infections caused by viruses are very common, causing high rates of mobility and mortality. There are few studies that relate to HBD2 and viral infection, and some of them are presented in the following paragraphs.

9.1 Influenza virus

The influenza virus belongs to the Orthomyxoviridae family and renders acute respiratory infection affecting mainly children and adults. It is an RNA virus, enveloped and has the ability to mutate rapidly, causing epidemics and pandemics [136].

Influenza virus induces the production of HBD2 in the epithelial cells of the respiratory tract *in vivo* and *in vitro* [137]. In the *in vitro* study with infected MDCK cells with influenza virus, recombinant murine β-defensin-2 prevents infection by blocking the entry of the virus. The lungs of murine model infected with influenza virus showed an increased expression of β-defensin and therefore confer protection against infection [21, 138].

9.2 Respiratory syncytial virus (VSR)

This virus belongs to the family Paramyxoviridae and affects principally infants, young children and older adults causing bronchiolitis and pneumonia. VSR has a high rate of morbidity and mortality having RNA enveloped virus of negative sense. There are no vaccines available and only fewer antivirals available which have been seen ineffective [22, 139].

The human lung cells (A549) infected with RSV expressed HBD2 [140]. The expression of the peptide depends on the activation of NF-kB and the action of TNF produced by the virus. The elimination of the virus is due to damage to the membrane.

9.3 Adenovirus

The adenoviruses belong to the Adenoviridae family; 51 serotypes divided into six species have been recognized (HAd A-F). Species B, C and E produce respiratory infections. Adenoviruses are double-stranded linear DNA viruses, lack envelope and replicate in the nucleus, and their genome has a size of 36 kb. These viruses spread rapidly in closed environments such as military camps, orphanages, boarding schools and prisons. The acute respiratory infections are transmitted mainly by aerosols and by direct inoculation through fingers. Although this disease is benign and with little severity, the infection might be severe in immunosuppressed patients afflicted with HIV and with kidney transplants. The HBD2 inactivates the infection for adenovirus *in vitro*; the mechanisms of action are not yet known due to lack of *in vivo* studies [140].

9.4 Rhinovirus

The rhinovirus is the main cause of the common cold belonging to Picornaviridae family. They are small, single-chained, naked RNA viruses. Respiratory infections caused by rhinoviruses are associated with asthma exacerbations in children and adults. Rhinovirus infection in the A549 cells (human lung cells) and bronchial epithelial cells induces the expression of HBD2. The virus replication appears essential for the expression of peptide [141].

10. Conclusions

Initially, β-defensin-2 was considered an antimicrobial peptide. The advance in the study of these molecules has made it possible to know that β-defensin-2 is a peptide with multiple functions. However, its role in the pathology of respiratory diseases is unclear. During the infectious processes of the respiratory epithelium, HBD2 is expressed by the effect of the infection, and it has been described that it may be closely associated with the severity of the disease. The study of HBD2 during viral respiratory infections is unclear, so it is necessary to continue investigating the role of this molecule in the immune response activated by viral infections.

Author details

Dora Patricia Rosete Olvera and Carlos Cabello Gutiérrez*
Department of Virology and Mycology, National Institute of Respiratory Diseases, Ismael Cosío Villegas, Ciudad de México, Mexico

*Address all correspondence to: carloscginer@gmail.com

References

[1] Gallo RL, Murakami M, Ohtake T, Zaiou M. Biology and clinical relevance of naturally occurring antimicrobial peptides. The Journal of Allergy and Clinical Immunology. 2002;**110**:823-831. DOI: 10.1067/mai.2002.129801

[2] Diamond G, Beckloff N, Ryan LK. Host defense peptides in the oral cavity and the lung: Similarities and differences. Journal of Dental Research. 2008;**87**:915-927. DOI: 10.1177/154405910808701011

[3] Hazlett L, Wu M. Defensins in innate immunity. Cell and Tissue Research. 2011;**343**:175-188. DOI: 10.1007/s00441-010-1022-4

[4] Schröder JM, Harder J. Human beta-defensin-2. The International Journal of Biochemistry & Cell Biology. 1999;**31**:645-651

[5] Harder J, Siebert R, Zhang Y, Matthiesen P, Christophers E, Schlegelberger B, et al. Mapping of the gene encoding human β-defensin-2 (DEFB2) to chromosome region 8p22-p23. Genomics. 1997;**46**:472-475

[6] McNamara NA, Van R, OR T, Fleiszigo SMJ. Surface epithelia express mRNA for human beta defensin-2. Experimental Eye Research. 1999;**69**:483-490

[7] Garreis F, Schlorf T, Worlitzsch D, Steven P, Bräuer L, Jäger K, et al. Roles of human α-defensins in innate immune defense at the ocular surface: Arming and alarming corneal and conjunctival epithelial cells. Histochemistry and Cell Biology. 2010;**134**:59-73. DOI: 10.1007/s00418-010-0713-y

[8] Bals R, Goldman MJ, JM W. Mouse β-defensin 1 is a salt-sensitive antimicrobial peptide present in epithelia of the lung and urogenital tract. Infection and Immunity. 1998;**66**:1225-1232

[9] Doss M, White MR, Tecle T, Hartshorn KL. Human defensins and LL-37 in mucosal immunity. Journal of Leukocyte Biology. 2010;**87**:79-92. DOI: 10.1189/jlb.0609382

[10] Garcia-Lopez G, Flores-Espinosa P, Zaga-Clavellina V. Tissue-specific human beta-defensins (HBD) 1, HBD2, and HBD3 secretion from human extra-placental membranes stimulated with *Escherichia coli*. Reproductive Biology and Endocrinology. 2010;**8**:146

[11] Gursoy UK, Könönen E. Understanding the roles of gingival beta defensins. Journal of Oral Microbiology. 2012;**4**:1-10. DOI: 10.34021jom.V410.15127

[12] Hertz CJ, Wu Q, Porter EM, Zhang YJ, Weismüller KH, Godowski PJ, et al. Activation of toll-like receptor 2 on human tracheobronchial epithelial cells induces the antimicrobial peptide human β-defensin-2. Journal of Immunology. 2003;**171**:6820-6826. DOI: 10.4049/jimmunol.171.12.6820

[13] Hill DR, Kessler SP, Rho HK, Cowman MK, De la Motte CA. Specific-sized hyaluronan fragments promote expression of human β-defensins-2 in intestinal epithelium. The Journal of Biological Chemistry. 2012;**287**:30610-30624. DOI: 10.1074/jbc.M112.356238

[14] Kesting MR, Mueller C, Wagenpfeil S, Stoeckelhuber M, Steiner T, Bauer F, et al. Quantitative comparison of the expression of antimicrobial peptides in the oral mucosa and extraoral skin. British Journal of Oral and Maxillofacial Surgery. 2012;**50**:447-453. DOI: 10.1016/j.bjoms.2011.07.006

[15] Auvynet C, Rosenstein Y. Multifunctional host defense

peptides: Antimicrobial peptides, the small yet big players in innate and adaptive immunity. FEBS Journal. 2009;**276**:6497-6508. DOI: 10.1111/j.1742-4658.2009.07360.x

[16] Mattar EH, Almehdar HA, Yacouba HA, Uversky WN, Redwan EM. Antimicrobial potentials and structural disorder of human and animal defensins. Cytokine & Growth Factor Reviews. 2016;**28**:95-111

[17] Semple F, Dorin JR. Defensins: Multifunctional modulators of infection, inflammation and more. Journal of Innate Immunity. 2012;**4**: 337-348. DOI: 10.1159/000336619

[18] Varshney J, Varshney H. Allergic rhinitis: An overview. Indian Journal of Otolaryngology and Head & Neck Surgery. 2015;**67**:143-149. DOI: 10.1007/s12070-015-0828-5

[19] Ooi CY, Pang T, Leach ST, Katz T, Day AS, Jaffe A. Fecal human β-defensin-2 in children with cystic fibrosis: Is there a diminished intestinal innate immune response? Digestive Diseases and Sciences. 2015;**60**: 2946-2952. DOI: 10.1007/s10620-015-3842-2

[20] Rivas SBT, Torres Rojas M, Bobadilla Lozoya K, Sada Díaz E. Papel de las células epiteliales en la respuesta inmune del pulmón. Revista del Instituto Nacional de Enfermedades Respiratorias. 2005;**18**:321-326

[21] Findlay EG, Currie SM, Davidson DJ. Cationic host defense peptides: Potential as antiviral therapeutics. BioDrugs. 2013;**27**:479-493. DOI: 10.1007/s40259-013-0039-0

[22] Ding J, Chou YY, Chang TL. Defensins in viral infections. Journal of Innate Immunity. 2009;**1**:413-420. DOI: 10.1159/000226256

[23] Duits LA, Nibbering PH, Van Strijen E, Vos JB, Mannesse-Lazeroms SPG, Van Sterkenburg MAJA, et al. Rhinovirus increases human β-defensin-2 and -3 mRNA expression in cultured bronchial epithelial cells. FEMS Immunology and Medical Microbiology. 2003;**38**:59-64. DOI: 10.1016/S0928-8244 (03) 00106-8

[24] Dhople V, Krukemeyer A, Ramamoorthy A. The human beta-defensin-3, an antibacterial peptide with multiple biological functions. Biochimica et Biophysica Acta. 2006;**1758**:1499-1512

[25] Chen H, Xu Z, Peng L, Fang X, Yin X, Xu N, et al. Recent advances in the research and development of human defensins. Peptides. 2006;**27**:931-940. DOI: 10.1016/j.peptides.2005.08.018

[26] De Y, Biragyn A, Kwak LW, Oppenheim JJ. Mammalian defensins in immunity: More than just microbicidal. Trends in Immunology. 2002;**23**:291-296

[27] Mallow EB, Harrisi A, Salzman N, Russell JP, DeBerardinis RJ, Ruchelli E, et al. Human enteric defensins. human enteric defensins. Gene structure and developmental expression. The Journal of Biological Chemistry. 1996;**271**:4038-4045

[28] Izadpanah A, Gallo RL. Antimicrobial peptides. Journal of the American Academy of Dermatology. 2005;**52**:381-390. DOI: 10.1016/j.jaad.2004.08.026

[29] Singh PK, Jia HP, Wiles K, Hesselberth J, Liu L, Conway BD, et al. Production of β-defensins by human airway epithelia. Proceedings of the National Academy of Sciences of the United States of America. 1998;**95**:14961-14966

[30] Braff MH, Bardan A, Nizet V, Gallo RL. Cutaneous defense mechanisms by antimicrobial peptides. The Journal of Investigative Dermatology. 2005;**125**:9-13

[31] Chen PH, Fang SY. Expression of human β-defensin-2 in human nasal mucosa. European Archives of Oto-Rhino-Laryngology. 2004;**261**:238-241. DOI: 10.1007/s00405-003-0682-z

[32] Guaní GE, Santos-Mendoza T, Lugo-Reyes SO, Terán LM. Antimicrobial peptides: General overview and clinical implications in human health and disease. Clinical Immunology. 2010;**135**:1-11. DOI: 10.1016/j.clim.2009.12.004

[33] Jarczak J, Kosciuczuk EM, Lisowski P, Strzałkowska N, Józwik A, Horbanczuk J, et al. Defensins: Natural component of human innate immunity. Human Immunology. 2013;**74**:1069-1079

[34] Schutte BC, Mitros JP, Bartlett JA, Walters JD, Jia HP, Welsh MJ, et al. Discovery of five conserved β-defensin gene clusters using a computational search strategy. PNAS. 2002;**99**:2129-2133

[35] Bruhn O, Grötzinger J, Cascorbi I, Jung S. Antimicrobial peptides and proteins of the horse-insights into a well-armed organism. Veterinary Research. 2011;**42**:1-22

[36] Corrales GL, Ortiz E, Castañeda-Delgado J, Rivas-Santiago B, Corzo G. Bacterial expression and antibiotic activities of recombinant variants of human β-defensins on pathogenic bacteria and *M. tuberculosis*. Protein Expression and Purification. 2013;**89**:33-43

[37] Machado LR, Ottolini B. An evolutionary history of defensins: A role for copy number variation in maximizing host innate and adaptive immune responses. Frontiers in Immunology. 2015;**6**:1-9. DOI: 10.3389/fimmu.2015.00115

[38] Hans M, Hans VM. Epithelial antimicrobial peptides: Guardian of the oral cavity. International Journal of Peptides. 2014;**2014**:370297. DOI: 10.1155/2014/370297

[39] Bakaletz L. Innate Immunity and the role of defensins in otitis media. Current Allergy and Asthma Reports. 2011;**11**:499-507. DOI: 10.1007/s11882-011-0223-6

[40] Taylor K, Clarke DJ, McCullough B, Chin W, Seo E, Yang D, et al. Analysis and separation of residues Important for the chemoattractant and antimicrobial activities of β-defensin-3. The Journal of Biological Chemistry. 2008;**283**:6631-6639

[41] Schneider JJ, Unholzer A, Schaller M, Schäfer KM, Korting HC. Human defensins. Journal of Molecular Medicine. 2005;**83**:587-595. DOI: 10.1007/s00109-005-0657-1

[42] Lan H, Chen H, Chen LC, Wang BB, Sun L, Ma YM, et al. The first report of a pelecaniformes defensin cluster: Characterization of β-defensin genes in the crested ibis based on BAC libraries. Scientific Reports;**4**:1-10. DOI: 10.1038/srep06923

[43] Tsutsumi IY, Nagaoka I. NF-kB-mediated transcriptional regulation of human β-defensin-2 gene following lipopolysaccharide stimulation. Journal of Leukocyte Biology. 2002;**71**:154-162. DOI: 10.4049/jimmunol.170.8.4226

[44] Frew L, Stock SJ. Antimicrobial peptides and pregnancy. Reproduction. 2011;**141**:725-735. DOI: 10.1530/REP-10-0537

[45] Ganz T. Defensins: Antimicrobial peptides of vertebrates. Comptes Rendus Biologies. 2004;**327**:539-549. DOI: 10.1016/j.crvi.2003.12.007

[46] McDermott AM. The role of antimicrobial peptides at the ocular surface. Ophthalmic Research. 2009;**41**:60-75

[47] Abiko Y, Saitoh M, Nishimura M, Yamazaki M, Sawamura D, Tohru Kaku D. Role of β-defensins in oral epithelial health and disease. Medical Molecular Morphology. 2007;**40**:179-184. DOI: 10.1007/s00795-007-0381-8

[48] Bals R, Wang X, Wu Z, Freeman T, Bafna V, Zasloff M, et al. Human β-defensin-2 is a salt-sensitive peptide antibiotic expressed in human lung. The Journal of Clinical Investigation. 1998;**102**:874-880

[49] Jang BC, Ki-Jo L, Ji-Hye P, Young-Kyu K, Sang-Woo S, Sang-Chan K, et al. Up-regulation of human β-defensin-2 by interleukin-1β in A549 cells: Involvement of PI3K, PKC, p38 MAPK, JNK, and NF-KB. Biochemical and Biophysical Research Communications. 2004;**320**:1026-1033. DOI: 10.1016/j.bbrc.2004.06.049

[50] Moon SK, Lee HY, Pan H, Takeshita T, Park R, Cha K, et al. Synergistic effect of interleukin 1 alpha on nontypeable *Haemophilus influenzae*-induced up-regulation of human beta-defensin 2 in middle ear epithelial cells. BMC Infectious Diseases. 2006;**6**:1-10

[51] Méndez SP, Miranda E, Trejo A. *Mycobacterium bovis* Bacillus Calmette-Guérin (BCG) stimulates human β-defensin-2 gene transcription in human epithelial cells. Cellular Immunology. 2006;**239**:61-66. DOI: 10.1016/j.cellimm.2006.04.001

[52] Martin E, Ganz T, Lehrer RI. Defensins and other endogenous peptide antibiotics of vertebrates. Journal of Leukocyte Biology. 1995;**58**:128-136

[53] Becker MN, Diamond G, Verghese MW, Randell SH. CD14-dependent Lipopolysaccharide-induced β-Defensin-2 expression in human tracheobronchial epithelium. The Journal of Biological Chemistry. 2000;**275**:29731-27936

[54] Lua Z, Kima KA, Suicoa MA, Shutoa T, Lib JD, Kaia H. MEF up-regulates human β-defensin-2 expression in epithelial cells. FEBS Letters. 2004;**561**:117-121. DOI: 10.1016/S0014-5793 (04) 00138-3

[55] Mineshiba J, Myokai F, Mineshiba F, Matsuura K, Nishimura F, Takashiba S. Transcriptional regulation of β-defensin-2 by lipopolysaccharide in cultured human cervical carcinoma (HeLa) cells. FEMS Immunology and Medical Microbiology. 2005;**45**:37-44. DOI: 10.1016/j.femsim.2005.01.008

[56] Harder J, Meyer-Hoffert U, Teran LM, Schwichtenberg L, Bartels J, Maune S, et al. Mucoid *Pseudomonas aeruginosa*, TNFa, and IL-1 b, but not IL-6, induced human β-defensin-2 in respiratory epithelia. American Journal of Respiratory Cell and Molecular Biology. 2000;**22**:714-721

[57] Scharf S, Hippenstiel S, Flieger A, Suttorp N, N'Guessan PD. Induction of human -defensin-2 in pulmonary epithelial cells by *Legionella pneumophila*: Involvement of TLR2 and TLR5, p38 MAPK, JNK, NF-kB, and AP-1. American Journal of Physiology. Lung Cellular and Molecular Physiology. 2010;**298**:L687-L695. DOI: 10.1152/ajplung.00365.2009

[58] Kim YJ, Shin HS, Lee JH, Jung YW, Kim HB, Ha UH. Pneumolysin-mediated expression of β-defensin-2 is coordinated by p38 MAP kinase-MKP1 in human airway cells. Journal of Microbiology. 2013;**51**:194-199. DOI: 10.1007/s12275-013-2579-x

[59] Mendez SP. Role of antimicrobial peptides in host defense against mycobacterial infections. Peptdes. 2008;**29**:1836-1841

[60] Semlali A, Witoled C, Alanazi M, Rouabhia M. Whole cigarette smoke increased the expression of TLRs, HBDs, and proinflammory cytokines by

human gingival epithelial cells through different signaling pathways. PLoS One. 2012;**7**(12):e52614. DOI: 10.1371/journal.pone.0052614

[61] Pace E, Ferraro M, Minervini MI, Vitulo P, Pipitone L, Chiappara G, et al. Beta defensin-2 is reduced in central but not in distal airways of smoker COPD patients. PLoS One. 2012;**7**:1-8. DOI: 10.1371/journal.pone.0033601

[62] Aguilar JW, Zapata W, Caruz A, Rugeles MT. High transcript levels of vitamin D receptor are correlated with higher mRNA expression of human beta defensins and IL-10 in mucosa of HIV-1-exposed seronegative individuals. PLoS One. 2013;**8**:1-9. DOI: 10.1371/journal.pone.0082717

[63] Pinheiro DP, Machado MCC. Antimicrobial peptides: Clinical relevance and therapeutic implications. Peptides. 2012;**36**:308-314

[64] Huang FC. De Novo sphingolipid synthesis is essential for *Salmonella*-induced autophagy and human beta-defensin 2 expressions in intestinal epithelial cells. Gut Pathogens. 2016;**8**:1-11. DOI: 10.1186/s13099-016-0088-2

[65] Chung WO, Hansen SR, Rao D, Dale BA. Expression increases epithelial antimicrobial peptide protease-activated receptor signaling. Journal of Immunology. 2004;**173**:5165-5170. DOI: 10.4049/jimmunol.173.8.5165

[66] Jenssen H, HamilL P, Hancock REW. Peptide antimicrobial agents. Clinical Microbiology Reviews. 2006;**19**:491-511. DOI: 10.1128/CMR.00056-05

[67] Raj PA, Dentino AR. Current status of defensins and their role in innate and adaptive immunity. FEMS Microbiology Letters. 2002;**206**:9-18

[68] Reddy KVR, Yedery RD, Aranha C. Antimicrobial peptides: Premises and promises. International Journal of Antimicrobial Agents. 2004;**24**:536-547. DOI: 10.1016/j.ijantimicag.2004.09.005

[69] Lai Y, Gallo RL. AMPed up immunity: How antimicrobial peptides have multiple roles in immune defense. Trends in Immunology. 2009;**30**:131-141. DOI: 10.1016/j.it.2008.12.003

[70] McDermott AM, Redfern RL, Zhang B, Pei Y, Huang L, ProskeInvest RJ. Defensin expression by the cornea: Multiple signaling pathways mediate IL-1β stimulation of hBD-2 expression by human corneal epithelial cells. Investigative Ophthalmology & Visual Science. 2003;**44**:1859-1865

[71] Rohrl J, De Y, Oppenheim JJ, Hehlgans T. Human β-defensin-2 and 3 and their mouse orthologs induce chemotaxis through interaction with CCR2. Journal of Immunology. 2010;**184**:6688-6694. DOI: 10.4049/jimmunol.0903984

[72] Niyonsaba F, Iwabuchi K, Matsuda H, Ogawa H, Nagaoka I. Epithelial cell-derived human β-defensin-2 acts as chemotaxin for mast cells through a pertussis toxin-sensitive and phospholipase C-dependent pathway. International Immunology. 2002;**14**:421-426

[73] Bhat S, Song YH, Lawye C, Milner SM. Modulation of the complement system by human β-defensin 2. Journal of Burns and Wounds. 2007;**5**:75-86

[74] Zimmer A, Hobkirk J, Mohamed F, Browning MJ, Stover CM. One the functional overlap between complement and anti-microbial peptides. Frontiers in Immunology. 2015;**5**:1-10. DOI: 10.3399/fimmu.2014.00689

[75] Al Rayahi IAM, Sanyi RHH. The overlapping roles of antimicrobial peptides and complement in recruitment and activation of tumor associated inflammatory cells. Frontiers

and Inmmunology. 2015;**6**:1-5. DOI: 10.3389/fimmu.2015.00002

[76] Dong H, Lv Y, Zhao D, Barrow P, Zhou X. Defensins: The case for their use against Mycobacterial infections. Journal of Immunology Research. 2016;Pages 1-9. Article ID: 7515687. http://dx.doi.org/10.1155/2016/7515687

[77] Brown KL, Hancock REW. Cationic host defense (antimicrobial) peptides. Current Opinion in Immunology. 2006;**18**:24-30. DOI: 10.1016/j.coi.2005.11.004

[78] Donnarumma G, Paoletti I, Buommino E, Iovene MA, Tudisco L, Cozza V, et al. Anti-inflammatory effects of moxifloxacin and human β-defensin 2 associations in human lung epithelial cell line (A549) stimulated with lipopolysaccharide. Peptides. 2007;**28**:286-292. DOI: 10.1016/j.peptides.2007.09.009

[79] Beard JA, Beardena A, Strikera R. Vitamin D and the anti-viral state. Journal of Clinical Virology. 2011;**50**:194-200. DOI: 10.1016/j.jcv.2010.12.006

[80] McNally JD, Sampson M, Matheson LA, Hutton B, Little J. Vitamin D receptor (VDR) polymorphisms and severe RSV bronchiolitis: A systematic review and meta-analysis. Pediatric Pulmonology. 2014;**49**:790-799. DOI: 10.1002/ppul.22877

[81] Weithauser A, Bobbert P, Antoniak S, Böhm A, Rauch BH, Klingel K, et al. Protease-activated receptor-2 regulates the innate immune response to viral infection in a coxsackievirus B3–induced myocarditis. Journal of the American College of Cardiology 2013; **62**:1737-1745

[82] Dommisch H, Chung WO, Rohani MG, Williams D, Rangarajan M, Curtis MA, et al. Protease-activated receptor 2 mediates human beta-defensin 2 and CC chemokine ligand 20 mRNA expression in response to proteases secreted by *Porphyromonas gingivalis*. Infection and Immunity. 2007;**75**:4326-4333. DOI: 10.1128/IAI.00455-07

[83] Jang BC, Lim KJ, Choi IH, Suh MH, Park JG, Mun KC, et al. Triptolide suppresses interleukin-1-β-induced human β-defensin-2 mRNA expression through inhibition of transcriptional activation of NF-κB in A549 cells. International Journal of Molecular Medicine. 2007;**19**:757-763

[84] Griffin S, Taggart CC, Greene CM, O'Neill S, McElvaney NG. Neutrophil elastase up-regulates human β-defensin-2 expression in human bronchial epithelial cells. FEBS Letters. 2003;**546**:233-236. DOI: 10.1016/S0014-5793 (03) 00577-5

[85] Fehlbaum P, Rao M, Zasloff M, Anderson GM. An essential amino acid induces epithelial β-defensin expression. PNAS. 2000;**97**:12723-12728

[86] Gariboldi S, Palazzo M, Zanobbio L, Selleri S, Sommariva M, Sfondrini L, et al. Low molecular weight hyaluronic acid increases the self-defense of skin epithelium by induction of β-defensin 2 via TLR2 and TLR4. Journal of Immunology. 2008;**181**:2103-2110. DOI: 10.4049/jimmunol.181.3.2103

[87] Lin L, Wen SH, Guo SZ, Su XY, Wu HJ, Chong L, et al. Role of SIRT1 in *β*-induced human β-defensin-2 and interleukin-8 expression in A549 cell. Molecular and Cellular Biochemistry. 2014;**394**:199-208. DOI: 10.1007/s11010-014-2095-2

[88] Mangoni ML, McDermott AM, Zasloff M. Antimicrobial peptides and wound healing: Biological and therapeutic considerations. Experimental Dermatology. 2016;**25**:67-173. DOI: 10.1111/exd.12929

[89] Suarez-Carmona M, Hubert P, Delvenne P, Herfs M. Defensins:

"Simple" antimicrobial peptides or broad-spectrum molecules? Cytokine & Growth Factor Reviews. 2015;**26**:361-370

[90] Ali RS, Falconer A, Ikram M, Bissett CE, Cerio R, Quinn AG. Expression of the peptide antibiotics human β-defensin-1 and human β-defensin-2 in normal human skin. The Journal of Investigative Dermatology. 2001;**117**:106-111

[91] Butmarc J, Yufit T, Carson P, Falanga V. First Human β-defensin-2 expression is increased in chronic wounds. Wound Repair and Regeneration. 2004;**12**:439-443

[92] Gonzalez-Curiel I, Trujillo V, Montoya-Rosales A, Rincon K, Rivas-Calderon B, DeHaro-Acosta J, et al. 1,25-Dihydroxyvitamin D3 induces LL-37 and HBD-2 production in keratinocytes from diabetic foot ulcers promoting wound healing: An *in vitro* Model. PLoS One. 2014;**9**:1-10

[93] Niyonsaba F, Ushio H, Nakano N, William N, Sayama K, Hashimoto K, et al. Antimicrobial peptides human β-defensins stimulate epidermal keratinocyte migration, proliferation and production of proinflammatory cytokines and chemokines. The Journal of Investigative Dermatology. 2007;**127**:594-604. DOI: 10.1038/sj.jid.5700599

[94] Baroni A, Donnarumma G, Paoletti L, Longanesi-Cattani I, Bifulco K, Tufano MA, et al. Antimicrobial human beta-defensin-2 stimulates migration, proliferation and tube formation of human umbilical vein endothelial cells. Peptides. 2009;**30**:267-272. DOI: 10.1016/j.peptides.2008.11.001

[95] Boniotto M, Jordan WJ, Eskdale J, Tossi A, Antcheva N, Crovella S, et al. Human β-defensin 2 induces a vigorous cytokine response in peripheral blood mononuclear cells. Antimicrobial Agents and Chemotherapy. 2006;**50**:1433-1441. DOI: 10.1128/AAC.50.4.1433-1441.2006

[96] Liu R, Zhang Z, Liu H, Hou P, Lang J, Wang S, et al. Human β-defensin 2 is a novel opener of Ca2+-activated potassium channels and induces vasodilation and hypotension in monkeys. Hypertension. 2013;**62**:415-425. DOI: 10.1161/HYPERTENSIONAHA.111.01076

[97] Diamond G, Kaiser V, Rhodes J, Russell JP, Bevins CL. Transcriptional regulation of β-defensin gene expression in tracheal epithelial cells. Infection and Immunity. 2000;**68**:113-119

[98] Hiratsuka T, Nakazato M, Date Y, Jun-ichi A, Minematsu T, Chino N, et al. Identification of human β-defensin-2 in respiratory tract and plasma and its increase in bacterial pneumonia. Biochemical and Biophysical Research Communications. 1998;**249**:943-947

[99] Ghosh SK, Gerken TA, Schneider KM, Feng Z, McCormick TS, Weinberg A. Quantification of human β-defensin-2 and -3 in body fluids: Application for studies of innate immunity. Clinical Chemistry. 2007;**53**:757-765

[100] Cakir E, Torun E, Gedik AH, Umutoglu T, Aktas EC, Topuz U, et al. Cathelicidin and human β-defensin 2 in bronchoalveolar lavage fluid of children with pulmonary tuberculosis. The International Journal of Tuberculosis and Lung Disease. 2013;**18**:671-675

[101] Harimurti K, Djauzi S, Witarto AB, Dewiasty E. Human β-defensin 2 concentration of respiratory tract mucosa in elderly patients with pneumonia and its associated factors. Acta Medica Indonesiana-Indonesian Journal of Internal Medicine. 2011;**43**(4):218-223

[102] Pacova H, Astl J, Martinek J. The pathogenesis of chronic inflammation and malignant transformation in the human upper airways: The role of beta-defensins, eNOS, cell proliferation and apoptosis. Histology and Histopathology. 2009;**24**:815-820

[103] Arimura Y, Ashitani JI, Yanagi S, Tokojima M, Abe K, Mukae Hand Nakazat M. Elevated serum defensins concentrations in patients with lung cancer. Anticáncer Reseach. 2004;**24**:4051-4058

[104] Liu S, He LR, Wang W, Wang GH, He ZY. Prognostic value of plasma human β-defensin 2 level on short-term clinical outcomes in patients with community-acquired pneumonia: A preliminary study. Respiratory Care. 2013;**58**:655-661. DOI: 10.4187/respcare.01827

[105] Dalcin D, Ulanova M. The role of human beta defensin 2 in *Pseudomonas aeruginosa* pulmonary infection in cystic fibrosis patients. Infectious Disease and Therapy. 2013;**2**:159-166. DOI: 10.1007/s40121-013-0015-5

[106] Claeys S, De Belder T, Holtappels G, Gevaert P, Verhasselt B, Van Cauwenberge P, et al. Human b-defensins and toll-like receptors in the upper airway. Allergy. 2003;**58**:748-753

[107] Dauletbaev N, Gropp R, Frye M, Loitsch S, Thomas-Otto-Friedrich, Joachim Bargon W. Expression of human beta defensin (HBD-1 and HBD-2) mRNA in nasal epithelia of adult cystic fibrosis patients, healthy individuals, and individuals with acute cold. Respiration. 2002;**69**:46-51

[108] Haarmann H, Steiner T, Schreiber F, Heinrich A, Zweigner J, Dje N'Guessan P, et al. The role and regulation of *Moraxella catarrhalis*-induced human betadefensin 3 expression in human pulmonary epithelial cells. Biochemical and Biophysical Research Communications. 2015;**467**:46-52

[109] Herr C, Beisswenger C, Hess C, Kandler K, Suttorp N, Welte T, et al. Suppression of pulmonary innate host defense in smokers. Thorax. 2009;**64**:144-149. DOI: 10.1136/thx.2008.102681

[110] Janssens W, Nuytten H, Dupont LJ, Van Eldere J, Vermeire S, Lambrechts D, et al. Genomic copy number determines functional expression of β-defensin 2 in airway epithelial cells and associates with chronic obstructive pulmonary disease. American Journal of Respiratory and Critical Care Medicine. 2010;**182**:163-169. DOI: 10.1164/rccm.200905-0767OC

[111] Liao Z, Dong J, Hu X, Wang T, Wan C, Li X, et al. Enhanced expression of human defensin 2 in peripheral lungs of patients with chronic obstructive pulmonary disease. Peptides. 2012;**38**:350-356

[112] Bogefors J, Mansson KA, Hockerfelt U, Lars-Olaf C. Reduced tonsillar expression of human β-defensin 1, 2 and 3 in allergic rhinitis. FEMS Immunology and Medical Microbiology. 2012;**65**:431-438. DOI: 10.1111/j.1574-695X.2012.00959.x

[113] Choi IJ, Chae-Seo R, Chul Hee L, Kim D-Y. Effect of allergic rhinitis on the expression of human β-defensin 2 in tonsils. Annals of Allergy, Asthma & Immunology. 2013;**110**:178-183

[114] Niyonsaba F, Kiatsurayanon C, Ogawa H. The role of human β-defensins in allergic diseases. Clinical & Experimental Allergy. 2016;**46**:1522-1530. DOI: 10.1111/cea.12843

[115] Ramnathan M, Lee WK, Spannhake EW. Th2 cytokines associated with chronic rhinosinusitis with polyps down-regulate the antmicorbial immunefunction of human sinonasal

epithelial cells. American Journal of Rhinology. 2008;**22**:115-121. DOI: 10.2500/ajr.2008.22.3136

[116] Hirschberg A, Kiss M, Kadocsa D, Polyanka H, Szabo K, Razga Z, et al. Different activations of toll-like receptors and antimicrobial peptides in chronic rhinosinusitis with or without nasal polyposis. European Archives of Oto-Rhino-Laryngology. 2016;**273**:1779-1788. DOI: 10.1007/s00405-015-3816-1

[117] Lee HY, Andalibi A, Webster P, Moon SK, Teufert K, Kang SH, et al. Antimicrobial activity of innate immune molecules against *Streptococcus pneumoniae, Moraxella catarrhalis* and nontypeable *Haemophilus influenza*. BMC Infectious Diseases. 2004;**4**:1-12

[118] Moon SK, Lee HY, Li JD, Nagura M, Kang SH, Chun YM, et al. Activation of a Src-dependent Raf–MEK1/2–ERK signaling pathway is required for IL-1a-induced upregulation of h-defensin 2 in human middle ear epithelial cells. Biochimica et Biophysica Acta. 2002;**1590**:41-51

[119] Bousquet J, Bousquet PJ, Godard P, Daures JP. The public health implications of asthma. Bulletin of the World Health Organization. 2005;**83**:548-554

[120] Yamaya M. Virus infection-induced bronchial asthma exacerbation. Pulmonary Medicine. 2012; Pages 1-14. Article ID: 834826. DOI: 10.1155/2012/834826

[121] Kwon JM, Shim JW, Kim DS, Jung HI, Park MS, Shim JY. Prevalence of respiratory viral infection in children hospitalized for acute lower respiratory tract diseases, and association of rhinovirus and influenza virus with asthma exacerbations. Korean Journal of Pediatrics. 2014;**57**:29-34

[122] Beisswenger C, Kandler K, Hess C, Garn H, Felgentreff K, Wegmann M, et al. Allergic airway inflammation inhibit pulmonary antibacterial host defenses. Journal of Immunology. 2006;**177**:1833-1837. DOI: 10.4049/jimmunol.177.3.1833

[123] Burd EM. Human papillomavirus and cervical cancer. Clinical Microbiology Reviews. 2003;**16**:1-17. DOI: 10.1128/CMR.16.1.1-17.2003

[124] Larson DA and and Derkay CS. Epidemiology of recurrent respiratory papillomatosis. APMIS. 2010;**118**:450-454. DOI: 10.1111/j.1600-0463.2010.02619.x

[125] Omland T, Akre H, Lie KA, Jebsen P, Sandvik L, Brøndbo K. Risk factors for aggressive recurrent respiratory papillomatosis in adults and juveniles. PLoS One. 2014;**9**(11):e113584. DOI: 10.1371/journal.pone.0113584

[126] Chong KT, Xiang L, Wang X, Jun EL, Xi L, Schweinfurth JM. High level expression of human epithelial β-defensins (hBD-1, 2 and 3) in papillomavirus induced lesions. Virology Journal. 2006;**3**(1-8):75. DOI: 10.1186/1743-422X-3-75

[127] Hiratsuka T, Mukae H, Iiboshi H, Ashitani J, Nabeshima K, Minematsu T, et al. Increased concentrations of human b-defensins in plasma and bronchoalveolar lavage fluid of patients with diffuse panbronchiolitis. Thorax. 2003;**58**:425-430

[128] Lonnroth K, Raviglione M. Global epidemiology of tuberculosis: Prospects for control. Seminars in Respiratory and Critical Care Medicine. 2008;**29**:481-491

[129] Shin DM, Jo EK. Antimicrobial peptides in innate immunity against mycobacteria. Immune Network. 2011;**11**:245-252

[130] Kisich KO, Heifets L, Higgins M, Diamond G. Antimycobacterial agent based on mRNA encoding

human β-defensin 2 enables primary macrophages to restrict growth of *Mycobacterium tuberculosis*. Infection and Immunity. 2001;**69**:2692-2699. DOI: 10.1128/IAI.69.4.2692-2699.2001

[131] Cervantes-Villagrana AR, Hernández-Pando R, Biragyn A, Castañeda-Delgado J, Bodogai M, Martínez-Fierro M, et al. Prime-boost BCG vaccination with DNA vaccines based in β-defensin-2 and mycobacterial antigens ESAT6 or Ag85B improve protection in a tuberculosis experimental model. Vaccine. 2013;**31**:676-684

[132] Rivas-Santiago B, Cervantes-Villagrana A, Sada E, Hernandez-Pandod R. Expression of beta defensin 2 in experimental pulmonary tuberculosis: Tentative approach for vaccine development. Archive of Medical Reseach. 2012;**3**:324-328

[133] Nickel D, Busch M, Mayer D, Hagemann B, Knoll V, Stenger S. Hypoxia triggers the expression of human β-defensin 2 and antimicrobial activity against *Mycobacterium tuberculosis* in human macrophages. Journal of Immunology. 2012;**188**: 4001-4007. DOI: 10.4049/jimmunol.1100976

[134] Klug-Micu GM, Stenger S, Sommer A, Liu PL, Krutzik SR, Modlin RL, et al. CD40 ligand and interferon-c induce an antimicrobial response against *Mycobacterium tuberculosis* in human monocytes. Immunology. 2013;**139**: 121-128. DOI: 10.1111/imm.12062

[135] Book M, Chen Q, Lehmann LE, Klaschik S, Weber S, Schewe JS, et al. Research inducibility of the endogenous antibiotic peptide β-defensin 2 is impaired in patients with severe sepsis. Critical Care. 2007;**11**:R19. DOI: 10.1186/cc5694

[136] Jiang Y, Wang Y, Kuang Y, Wang B, Li W, Gong T, et al. Expression of mouse beta-defensin-3 in MDCK cells and its anti-influenza-virus activity. Archives of Virology. 2009;**154**:639-647. DOI: 10.1007/s00705-009-0352-6

[137] Doss M, White MR, Tecle T, Gantz D, Crouch EC, Jung G, et al. Interactions of α-, β-, and θ-defensins with influenza A virus and surfactant protein D. Journal of Immunology. 2009;**182**:7878-7887. DOI: 10.4049/jimmunol.0804049

[138] Gong T, Jiang Y, Wang Y, De Y, Li W, Zhang Q, et al. Recombinant mouse beta-defensin 2 inhibits infection by influenza A virus by blocking its entry. Archives of Virology. 2010;**155**:491-498. DOI: 10.1007/s00705-010-0608-1

[139] Kota S, Sabbah A, Chang TH, Harnack R, Xiang Y, Meng X, et al. Role of human β-defensin-2 during tumor necrosis factor α/NF-kB-mediated innate antiviral response against human respiratory syncytial virus. The Journal of Biological Chemistry. 2008;**283**:22417-22429

[140] Galván Morales MA, Escobar Gutiérrez A, Rosete Olvera DP, Cabello Gutiérrez C. Effect of human beta defensin-2 in epithelial cell lines infected with respiratory viruses. Journal of Bioanalysis & Biomedicine. 2015;**7**:136-143. DOI: 10.4172/1948-593X.1000135

[141] Duits LA, Nibbering PH, van Strijen E, Vos JB, Mannesse LSPG, van Sterkenburg MAJA, et al. Rhinovirus increases human L-defensin-2 and -3 mRNA expression in cultured bronchial epithelial cells. FEMS Immunology and Medical Microbiology. 2003;**38**:59-64. DOI: 10.1016/S0928-8244 (03) 00106-8

Chapter 5

Immune Cell Activation: Stimulation, Costimulation, and Regulation of Cellular Activation

Suman Kapur and Anuradha Pal

Abstract

Opiate receptor (uOR) is expressed in central nervous system, gastrointestinal tract, male and female reproductive tissues, and immune cells. Morphine, a ligand for opioid receptor family, is known to activate the hypothalamic-pituitary-adrenal axis and release immunosuppressive glucocorticoids. Herein we present that minor changes, in the form of nonsynonymous single nucleotide polymorphisms, in μOR have cumulative impact on receptor-mediated signaling and functions of specific cell type(s). Significant reduction was seen in cells in M and S phases with coactivation of immune receptors with μOR. Flow cytometry-based experiments established a reduction in B and T lymphocytes, NK cells, and macrophages. Differences in types of immune cells were found to be significant to reduce immune response(s) mounted by GG(mutant allele)-bearing individuals. This is the first report on cross-talk between LPS-binding and μOR, explaining the reduction in the number of T and B cells after chronic opiate use and also the association of this impact on immunocytes with functional SNP, rs1799972/118G allele of OPRM1 gene as an explanation for the immune suppression in opiate users. Initially present lower cell titers can be further lowered by exogenous opiates and account for immunosuppression seen in chronic opiate users or after long-term treatment with opiate drugs for chronic pain.

Keywords: immune response activation, costimulation, cellular activation, opioid receptors

1. Immune system: a brief introduction

The immune system is a complex and highly developed system, yet its mission is simple: to seek and kill intruders. It is the body's defense system against infectious organisms and other invaders. The purpose of the immune system is to keep infectious microorganisms, such as bacteria, viruses, and fungi, out of the body, and to destroy any infectious microorganisms that do invade the body. Through a series of steps called the immune response, the immune system protects us against invading organisms. It is a network of cells, tissues, and organs working together to protect the body. The most important cell types involved in immune response are white blood cells, which come in two basic types that combine to seek out and destroy disease-causing organisms. Leukocytes are produced or stored in different locations in the body, like the thymus, spleen, bone marrow lymph nodes, and special deposits of lymphoid tissue (as in the gastrointestinal

Cell type	Location and function
Leukocytes	Derived from myeloid or lymphoid lineage, these are the main cells in immune system, which provide either innate or specific adaptive immunity. Myeloid cells include phagocytic, motile neutrophils, monocytes, and macrophages, providing the first-line defense against pathogens. Other myeloid cells involved in defense against parasites & in genesis of allergic reactions include eosinophils, basophils, & mast cells. Lymphocytes regulate the action of other leukocytes & generate specific responses to prevent chronic/recurrent infections [1]
B cells	In mammals, B cells mature in the bone marrow where as in birds, B cells mature in the bursa of Fabricius, a lymphoid organ first discovered by Chang and Glick [2]. They develop into antibody-secreting plasma cells. B cells express B cell receptors (BCRs) on their cell membrane that allows them to bind to specific antigen, against which it initiates a specific antibody response.
T cells	Originate in the bone marrow and mature in the thymus giving rise to helper, regulatory, cytotoxic T cells, or memory T cells. From the thymus, they migrate to peripheral tissues, blood, & lymphatic system. On stimulation, they secrete chemical messengers called cytokines, which stimulate the differentiation of B cells into antibody-producing cells also called plasma cells. Cytotoxic T cells in the presence of various cytokines bind to and kill infected and/or cancer cells.
T helper cells	Subset of T cells, found throughout the body, with especially high titers in lymphoid organs (lymph nodes and spleen), as well as the liver, lung, blood, and the intestinal tract. T helper TH or CD4+ T cells coordinate and regulate immunological responses. T_H cells mediate responses by secreting lymphokines that act on other cell types involved in mounting an immune response.
T cytotoxic cells	Subset of T cells, found throughout the body, with especially high titers in lymphoid organs (lymph nodes & spleen), as well as the liver, lung, blood, and the intestinal tract. T cytotoxic Tc or CD8+ T cells are involved in directly killing virus-infected cells, transplanted cells, and sometimes, eukaryotic parasites and tumor cells. CD8+ T cells have been shown to play a role in downregulating the immune response.
Natural Killer cells	NK cells are similar to Tc cells. They directly kill certain tumors such as melanomas, lymphomas and virus-infected cells- and clear herpes and cytomegalovirus-infected cells. In contrast to Tc cells, NK cells kill their target cells more effectively without the need for recognition of antigen in association with MHC molecules and are activated by secretions from T_H cells.
Macrophages	These are phagocytic cells and function as antigen-presenting cells (APCs) as they ingest foreign materials and present these to other members of the immune system such as T cells and B cells. Besides being the initiators of an immune response, they also act as immune modulators by secreting cytokines and can also be stimulated by lymphokines, to exhibit increased levels of phagocytosis.

Cell type	Location and function
Dendritic cells	Originate in the bone marrow and form another class of APCs. These are found in the lymphoid organs such as the thymus, lymph nodes, and spleen along with the bloodstream and other tissues. They function to capture and process antigens in lymphoid organs at the time of initiation of an immune response.
Neutrophils	These cells, which ingest, kill, and digest pathogens, are the most highly adherent and motile, phagocytic leukocytes; the first cell types to be recruited to acute inflammatory sites. Their functions are dependent on adherence molecule CD11b/CD18, or biochemical pathways, such as the respiratory burst associated with cytochrome b558.
Eosinophils	Defend against parasites and participate in hypersensitivity reactions. Their cytotoxicity is mediated through cytoplasmic granules containing eosinophilic basic and cationic proteins.
Basophils	Along with their tissue counterparts, mast cells produce cytokines required for defense against parasites and allergic inflammation. They display surface membrane receptors for IgE antibodies and possess cytoplasmic granules containing heparin and histamine. When cell-bound IgE antibodies are cross linked by antigens, the eosinophils degranulate releasing low-molecular weight vasoactive mediators (e.g., histamine), which mediate their biological effects.
Monocytes/macrophages	These are involved in phagocytosis and intracellular killing of microorganisms. Macrophages are differentiated monocytes, residing in the reticuloendothelial systems and act as antigen-presenting cells presenting processed peptides to T cells. They are recruited to inflammatory sites and further activated by exposure to certain cytokines, which potentiate their biologic functions.

Table 1.
Major cell types of adaptive immunity.

tract). These cells circulate through the body between the organs and nodes via lymphatic and blood vessels, and work in a coordinated manner to monitor the body for foreign invasions. A potent and active immune system is vital for staying healthy. The immune system differentiates between invaders and the body's own cells—when immune system is not able to differentiate between self and nonself, a reaction against "self" cells and molecules causes autoimmune disease. The immune system will remain active by getting enough sleep, exercise, and good nutrition.

Immune response leads to inflammation. The goal of inflammation is to get rid of the stimulus—both the disease-causing pathogens and/or neoplastic tissue. Significant steps involved in inflammation include recruitment of immune cells, interactions of these cells in the affected tissue and activation pattern of the interacting cells. The immune system continuously looks for pathogens, xenobiotics, and other nonself signals. Thus, the cell types of the immune system are incredibly dynamic and capable of upregulating processes required for handling these insults on a time scale of minutes to hours. Several cell types in this system are capable of activation to secrete cytokines, rapidly proliferate, or otherwise communicate to surrounding cells that there is a pathogen to consider. Upon clearance of the pathogen, the cell population must contract in a controlled manner. Furthermore, in some cell populations (e.g., T cells), a subset of cells is retained as long-lived memory cells to protect and prime the system for future insults. Researchers are increasingly focused on early events in immune cell activation, where the response to an inflammatory signal can be tuned to impact overall cell function. In areas such as immuno-oncology, increased activation is connected to improve cell expansion whereas in the field of immunosuppression, the converse is desired. Clinical successes in targeting the immune system for treating cancer have generated a resurgence of effort to harness the immune system more routinely for therapeutic intervention (**Table 1**).

2. Mechanism of activation of adapted immunity

Adaptive immune responses carried out by lymphocytes are of two broad classes:

- antibody responses carried out by B cells
- cell-mediated immune responses carried out by T cells

During an immune response, the B cells are activated to secrete immunoglobulins, which circulate in blood, permeate to other body fluids, and bind specifically to foreign antigen that stimulated their production in the first place. This binding inactivates viruses and microbial toxins by blocking their interaction with the host cells. Antibody binding also marks invading pathogens for destruction by phagocytic cells of the innate immune system [3].

Cell-mediated reactions depend on direct interactions between T lymphocytes and cells bearing the antigen that the T cells recognize. T cells are specialized to recognize foreign antigens as peptide fragments bound to proteins of the major histocompatibility complex (MHC). The cytotoxic T cells recognize any infected cells with the help of viral antigens displayed on the surface of the infected cells [1]. Other T lymphocytes that activate the cells they recognize are marked by the expression of the cell-surface molecule CD4 on helper T cells. The CD4 T lymphocytes can be divided into two subsets, which carry out different functions by defending the body particularly from bacterial infections. Bacteria phagocytosed by macrophages are destroyed in the lysosomes, which contain several enzymes and antimicrobial substances. The intracellular bacteria, as in case of tuberculosis (Mtb), survive, because the vesicles they occupy do not fuse with the lysosomes. These infections are modified by a subset of CD4 T cells, namely TH1 cells, which activate macrophages, induce fusion of lysosomes and phagocytic vesicles containing the bacteria, and at the same time stimulate other antibacterial mechanisms of the phagocyte. CD4+ T cells play critical role during Mtb infection by mediating protection, contributing to inflammation, and regulating immune response. Th1 and Th17 cells are the main effector CD4+ T cells during Mtb. Th1 cells release cytokines and chemokines that attract phagocytes to the site of infection and impart protection from Mtb by secreting IFN-γ and activating antimycobacterial action in macrophages.

T cells not only destroy intracellular pathogens by killing infected cells and by activating macrophages, but they also have a central role in the destruction of extracellular pathogens by activating B cells. This is the specialized role of the second subset of CD4 T cells called TH2 cells with special properties that can activate naive B lymphocytes. Most antigens require an accompanying signal from helper T cells before they can stimulate B cells to proliferate and differentiate into cells secreting antibody. Cytotoxic T cells and TH1 cells interact with antigens produced by pathogens that have infected the target cell or that have been ingested by it. Helper T cells, in contrast, recognize and interact with B cells that have bound and internalized foreign antigen by means of their surface immunoglobulin.

Antigen-specific activation of effector T cells is aided by coreceptors that distinguish between the two classes of MHC molecule—CD8 coreceptor bearing cytotoxic cells that binds MHC class I molecules, whereas TH1 and TH2 cells express the CD4 coreceptor with specificity for MHC class II molecules. The maturation of T cells into either CD8 or CD4 T cells reflects the type of T-cell receptor specificity that occurs during development, and the selection of T cells that can receive survival signals from self-MHC molecules. On recognizing their targets, the three types of T cell are stimulated to release different sets of effector molecules namely, cytokines, which play crucial role in the clonal expansion of lymphocytes as well as in the innate immune responses.

T cells are thus crucially important for both humoral and cell-mediated responses of adaptive immunity. The adaptive immune response seems to have engrafted specific antigen recognition by highly diversified receptors onto innate defense systems, which have a central role in the effector actions of both B and T lymphocytes. The vital role of adaptive immunity in fighting infection is illustrated by the immunodeficiency and/or autoimmune diseases and the problems caused by pathogens that succeed in evading or subverting an adaptive immune response. The antigen-specific suppression of adaptive immune responses is the goal of treatment for important human diseases involving inappropriate activation of lymphocytes, whereas the specific stimulation of an adaptive immune response is the basis of successful vaccination for several childhood infections.

3. Opioid receptor and immune function

As early as 1987, Jankovic and Maric [4] showed that the neuropeptides—methionine-enkephalin, and leucine-enkephalin, exhibit a protective action against anaphylactic shock in rats sensitized to ovalbumin. Subsequent studies have shown that enkephalins can act both as suppressors and potentiators of immune response in a dose-dependent manner. Animal studies, where nutritional status, environmental influences, history of drug abuse, and genetic variability can be controlled more easily, have shown that morphine treatment results in significant immune deficits. Chronic morphine use has been shown to result in severe immunosuppression, posing as a significant risk factor for opportunistic infection [5], and this finding is also supported by epidemiological studies that show an increased prevalence of opportunistic infections in opiate users [6]. Chronic morphine has been shown to effect early reactions of innate immunity and later responses of adaptive immunity against microbes [7]. In addition, morphine has also been shown to affect the brain-immune axis by an IL-1β-dependent pathway [8]. Various studies support the idea that chronic morphine exposure in vivo attenuates lymphocyte proliferation [9], NK cell cytotoxicity [10], antibody and serum hemolysin formation [11], and phagocytic properties of peripheral mononuclear leukocytes [12]. Morphine exposure has also been shown to increase mortality of infected mice [12–14]. Novick et al. [15] showed that long-term abuse of opiates results in impaired NK cell activity and altered CD4+

and CD8+ T cell numbers. In animal models, parenteral use of opiates was shown to inhibit mitogenic and effector cell responses in both B and T cells [9, 16].

3.1 Opioid receptors in various immune cell types and their functional implications

Molecular biology studies have shown that immune cells differentially express opioid receptors (OR), and morphine affects their development, differentiation, and function [17]. Binding sites and protein expression for delta (δ) and kappa (κ) subclasses of G protein-coupled ORs [18, 19], in addition to gene expression of δ, κ, and μ subclasses [20, 21], have been described in leukocytes. Chuang et al. [20] reported the presence of mRNA for the μOR in human T- and B-cell lines, CD4+ T cells, monocytes, macrophages and granulocytes. Retinoid receptor activation increases the expression of the μOR in U937 cells, a mononuclear cell line [22]. Mu (μ-), Kappa (κ-), and Delta (δ-) opioids have been shown to possess chemoattractant activity and induce the chemotaxis of both monocytes and neutrophils [23–28]. Simpkins et al. [24] and Van Epps and Saland [25] showed that opiates, acting through δ and μ subclasses of OR expressed on human monocytes and neutrophils, are capable of inhibiting subsequent migratory responses to chemokines, and that this process of heterologous desensitization/trans-deactivation is associated with phosphorylation of chemokine receptors. Grimm et al. [26] showed that phagocytes respond chemotactically, with a chemotaxis index 2- to 2.5-fold higher than controls, to met-enkephalin and morphine, and this chemotaxis was inhibited by the OR antagonist naloxone. Liu et al. [27] demonstrated that pretreatment with opioids, including morphine, heroin, met-enkephalin, the selective μ-agonist DAMGO, or the selective δ-agonist [D-Pen2, D-Pen5] enkephalin (DPDPE), leads to the inhibition of the chemotactic response of leukocytes to complement-derived chemotactic factors. They also affect the chemokines macrophage inflammatory protein (MIP-1α)/CCL3, RANTES/CCL5, monocyte chemotactic protein-1 (MCP-1)/CCL2, and IL-8/CXCL8 [28]. Many investigators choose to study the effects of morphine on immune function because morphine has clinical applications and shows good affinity for all three types of ORs. However, use of morphine as the opioid of choice has limited the ability to delineate, which type of OR mediates the given immunological response/s due to binding to all receptor types.

Existence of a low-affinity, naloxone-insensitive morphine binding site on human peripheral blood macrophages has also been reported [29]. Opioid alkaloids, such as morphine and the endogenous peptides, including β-endorphin and dynorphin, directly modulate the function of lymphocytes and other cells involved in host defense and immunity, ORs preferentially bind to the (−)-enantiomer of most opioid alkaloids, for example, ORs will bind the antagonist (−)-naloxone but not (+)-naloxone [30].

3.2 Immunosuppression mediated by opiates

The role of opiate drugs in suppressing a variety of immunological endpoints such as proliferation, functions and responses of both T and B cells, and attenuation of the cytokine system has been studied extensively [31, 32]. Opiate drug administration has also been reported to suppress movement and number of white blood cells [33, 34]. Heroin use has been documented to depress E-rosette formation indicating clinical immune suppression [35]. Long-term use of opiate drugs has been reported to depress T cell reactivity and cause a loss of T helper (T_H) cells [36, 37], reduces T helper/T cytotoxic cell ratios, and decreases T helper cell function [38–41]. Use of opiate drugs produces atrophy of lymphoid organs, decreases lymphoid content, and alters antigen-specific antibody production [42, 43]. Opiate addiction induces immunonutritional deficiencies [44, 45] and impairs immunoglobulin synthesis and function [46]. Naik et al. [47] showed a decrease of IgA levels and increase of IgG levels in Indian opiate users as compared to nonusers. Opioids bind directly on immune cells and modulate the function of these cells and also bind to classical ORs in the CNS, causing the release of catecholamines and/or steroids, which in turn also affect the immune cells. At the same time, morphine is known to activate the hypothalamic-pituitary-adrenal axis and release glucocorticoids, which are immunosuppressive in their own capacity [48].

3.3 Impact of functional polymorphism in OPRM1 gene on cell function

Several studies suggest that immune cells contain μORs along with existence of morphine binding sites differing from classical μORs, and measurements of the mRNAs that encode the neuronal types of OR show low levels of receptor mRNA in immune cells [49]. μOR is known to depict a total of 43 variants within coding and noncoding regions of the *OPRM1* gene, and 52 different haplotypes were predicted in the subgroup of African Americans. These haplotypes were classified by similarity clustering into functionally related categories, and one of these was significantly more frequent in substance-dependent individuals, viz. [−1793T-A, −1699insT, −1320A-G, −111C-T, +17C-T (+118A-G)], which was associated with substance dependence [50]. Studies evaluating the effects of 118A > G SNP on the intracellular signaling cascades resulting from μ-OR activation have shown conflicting results. Both DAMGO and morphine were twofold more potent in inhibiting calcium channel currents in sympathetic neurons transfected with the 118G allele than in neurons expressing the wild-type receptors [51]. However, Kroslak et al. [52] showed in HEK293 and AV-12 cells that stable expression of the 118G variant was associated with decreased agonist-mediated cyclic adenosine monophosphate (cAMP) signaling for morphine, methadone, and DAMGO, but not for β-endorphin. These results suggest that cellular environment may influence the phenotype associated with the variant receptor. Deb et al. [53], using murine neuroblastoma Neuro 2 A cells stably transfected with cDNA containing 118G variant, studied the effect on PKA, ERK, and CREB activation and documented no upregulation of PKA activity but a differential response of ERK phosphorylation in comparison to 118A variant, following chronic morphine treatment. Zhang et al. [54] analyzed 87 human brain tissue samples derived from autopsies and performed in vitro experiments on Chinese hamster ovary (CHO) cells, to show that the amount of mRNA transcribed from the 118G allele was twofold lower than the mRNA derived from the 118A allele. The levels of variant protein were ten-fold lower compared with those of the wild-type receptor. They also showed that after transfection into CHO cells with a cDNA representing only the coding region of *OPRM1* and inhibition of transcription with actinomycin D, the mRNA turnover was same for 118A and 118G variants. An *in silico* study by Pang et al. [55] showed that the substitution of the A with G at position 118 of the *OPRM1* gene abolishes three transcription factor binding sites, while creating a novel exon splice enhancer as well as p53 and a zinc finger protein binding sites, predicting a direct effect of 118A > G on gene expression and on the processing of heterogeneous nuclear RNA into mature mRNA. Huang et al. [56] described the role of the 118A > G SNP in posttranslational mechanisms suggesting that N-glycosylation may affect receptor expression, since it plays an important role in correct folding of receptors in the endoplasmic reticulum and, hence, their sorting from the endoplasmic reticulum to the plasma membrane. Huang et al. [56] also showed that the variant receptor had lower relative molecular mass than the wild-type one, which may be explained by a differential glycosylation status between the two receptors. Pulse-chain (or chase) experiments revealed that the half-life of the mature form of the variant receptor (~12 h) was shorter than that of the wild-type receptor (~28 h) showing its effect on protein stability. Thus, several lines of evidence suggest that the 118G variant may affect *OPRM1* gene expression in addition to mRNA translation, posttranslational processing, or turnover of the μ-opioid receptor protein, which can all effect signaling pathway/s.

3.4 Epigenetics of OPRM1 gene and its impact on cell function

Human genome has about 45,000-C-phosphate-G-(CpG) islands, many in the promoter regions of genes. The CpG islands are located upstream of the transcription start site to within the first exon [57]. Nielsen et al. [58] and Chorbov et al. [59] reported that in DNA obtained from peripheral lymphocytes, two of 16 CpG sites in a region of *OPRM1* gene promoter had significantly higher methylation in former heroin addicts than in controls. These two CpG sites are located in binding sites for the potential Sp1 transcription factor. Oertel et al. [60] showed that substitution of an A with a G at gene position +118 introduces a new CpG-methylation site at position +117, which leads to enhanced methylation of *OPRM1* gene resulting in decreased expression. Using m-fold software, Johnson et al. [61] showed that 118G variant demonstrated an altered folding that could affect mRNA stability. The epigenetic mechanism reported by Oertel et al. [60] impedes μ-OR upregulation in brain tissue, and they concluded that while in wild-type subjects, a reduced signaling efficiency associated with chronic heroin exposure was compensated for by an increased receptor density; this upregulation was absent in carriers of the 118G receptor variant due to diminished *OPRM1* mRNA transcription. The *OPRM1* 118A > G SNP variant not only reduces μ-OR signaling efficiency, but by a genetic-epigenetic interaction, also reduces OR expression and therefore, depletes the opioid system of a compensatory reaction to chronic exposure, providing evidence that a change in the genotype can cause a change in the epigenotype with major functional consequences.

3.5 Receptor-receptor interactions

Oligomerization is a general characteristic of cell membrane receptors that is shared by G protein-coupled receptors (GPCRs). GPCRs do not exist in isolation and interact with components of the bilayer, such as lipids and sterols, as well as with other GPCRs to form dimers and higher order oligomers, which are of functional significance as this affects the ligand binding and signaling properties of GPCRs [62, 63]. Recent studies of these complexes, both in vivo and in purified reconstituted forms, unequivocally support this contention for GPCRs [64]. A large number of direct binding assays indicating negative or positive cooperativity suggest clustering of GPCRs [65]. Mansoor et al. [66] reported that GPCRs can come together in the presence of lipids. Oligomerization and the two monomers comprising a GPCR dimer could be nonequivalent, thereby allowing more refined regulation of GPCR activity [66–68]. Thus, GPCR dimerization can be the result of the receptors forming heterodimers as well as homodimers [69], with many dimers displaying modified pharmacology [70], altered responsiveness to viral entry through GPCRs [71], or attenuated signaling [72]. Therefore, it is apparent that the oligomeric potential of GPCRs allows further diversification of their repertoire as a result of more complex ligand-receptor relationships than envisioned for monomeric receptors due to a more complex ligand-receptor relationship [64]. Although monomeric GPCRs can activate G proteins, the pentameric structure constituted by one GPCR homodimer and one heterotrimeric G protein may constitute the functional unit, and oligomeric entities can be viewed as multiples of dimers [73].

3.6 Interactions of opioid receptors

Fluorescence correlation spectroscopy (FCS) studies suggest that μ-opioid receptors exist primarily as dimers that oligomerize with δ-opioid receptors into tetramers [74]. High-resolution crystallographic structures of the μ-opioid by Manglik et al. [75] showed that they exist as parallel dimers and/or tetramers. Some TM domains have been observed more often than others. TM5 and TM6 residues constituted the main interfaces for the μ-opioid receptor crystallized dimers, with extensive contacts throughout the length of these TM helices in μ-opioid receptor dimers. The μ-opioid dimers also showed a second, less prominent symmetric interface, involving TM1, TM2, and helix 8 (H8; the helix adjacent to TM7 running along the internal membrane surface [75]). For GPCRs, the majority of crystal structures that are currently available refer to antagonist-bound (inactive) structures. The inferred dimeric interfaces may, therefore, depend on specific conformational states. Furthermore, the TM5-TM6 interface inferred by the crystal structure of μ-opioid dimers could preclude either monomer from properly coupling to G protein, because the agonist-induced receptor-G protein interaction depends on rearrangements of TM5 and TM6 within the seven-helical domain bundle, suggesting that different receptor conformations stabilized with different ligands may also promote different dimeric interfaces [75]. Huang et al. [76] suggested that the comparison of the differences in the interfaces observed from the crystallized structures of the antagonist-bound μ-opioid and chemokine CXCR4 receptors and the ligand-free β1-adrenoceptor suggest that the TM5 interface can partner in the interaction with TM4 or TM6, depending on the conformation of the receptor.

In δ-μ-OR heteromers, it was shown that binding and signaling by morphine or μ receptor agonists were potentiated by δ-OR antagonists, and reciprocally, binding and signaling by δ-OR agonists were potentiated by μ receptor selective antagonists [77, 78]. Studies carried out with the δ-opioid-cannabinoid CB1 receptor heteromer have also revealed allosteric modulations of cannabinoid CB1 receptor ligands on δ-OR ligand binding properties [79, 80]. They also showed that in recombinant systems expressing both receptors, as well as endogenous tissues, binding and consequently signaling by δ-OR could be potentiated by a low, nonsignaling dose of cannabinoid CB1 receptor agonist or a selective antagonist. In the δ-μ-OR heteromers, Gupta et al. [81] showed that morphine-induction increases heteromer abundance. Similarly, the δ-opioid-CB1 receptor heteromer increases in the brain after peripherally elicited neuropathic pain [79]. Studies by Zheng et al. [82] have revealed a complex interplay among cholesterol, palmitate, receptor dimerization, and G protein activation. They showed that reducing cholesterol levels or preventing palmitoylation of the μOR reduced receptor dimerization and Gα association. Additionally, preventing palmitoylation reduced the association of μOR with cholesterol, suggesting a functional complex of receptor, palmitate, and cholesterol. The authors also demonstrate that mutagenesis of the palmitoylated cysteine residue in μOR has no effect on ligand binding but decreased signaling efficiency, probably by impairing GPCR-G protein association. The same mutant had significantly reduced dimerization, and it was proposed that this was responsible for the reduced G protein coupling. Zhang et al. [83] demonstrated that the palmitate-free mutant associated more weakly with cholesterol. A model of the μOR dimer in which cholesterol and palmitate pack together to facilitate receptor dimerization reveals that cholesterol interactions contribute approximately 25% of the total interaction energy at the homodimer interface [82].

3.7 Receptor dimerization and immune cell stimulation and functioning

Chemokines are chemotactic cytokines that mediate their effects on leukocytes through a number of G protein-coupled, seven transmembrane-spanning (STM) receptors [84]. Specificity is provided by patterns of receptor and G protein expression, ligand potency, and levels of receptor desensitization. Interactions among receptors are mediated through a process known as receptor cross regulation, or heterologous desensitization [85]. Ali et al. [86] showed that thrombin receptor activation causes phosphorylation of several chemoattractant receptors, including the IL-8 receptor CXCR1, the C5a receptor, and the receptor for platelet-activating factor 3. Ben-Baruch et al. [87] have shown that homologous desensitization through phosphorylation of the IL-8 receptor CXCR2 occurs in response to its native ligands IL-8 and neutrophil-activating peptide (NAP)-2. Grimm et al. [28] showed that opiates, acting through δ and μ subclasses of opioid receptors expressed on human monocytes and neutrophils, are capable of inhibiting subsequent migratory responses to chemokines, and that this process of heterologous desensitization or trans-deactivation is associated with phosphorylation of chemokine receptors. Szabo et al. [88] showed that the chemotactic activities of both μ- and δ-OR are desensitized following activation of the chemokine receptors CCR5, CCR2, CCR7, and CXCR4 but not of CXCR1 or CXCR2 receptors. The inhibition of CCL3 and CCL5 responses following opioid pretreatment is consistent with the desensitization of either CCR1 or CCR5 or both. This receptor cross talk results in heterologous desensitization and phosphorylation of some of the chemokine receptors, which subsequently contribute to the immunosuppressive effects of the opioids.

4. Immune receptors and their function

Cells of the immune system intercommunicate by ligand-receptor interactions between cells and/or via secreted molecules called cytokines. Cytokines produced by lymphocytes are termed lymphokines (i.e., interleukins & interferon-γ), and those produced by monocytes and macrophages are termed monokines [89]. The

	T cells	B cells	NK cells	Monocytes/ macrophages
Antigen recognition	+	+	–	–
Antigen presentation	–	+	–	+
Antibody production	–	+	–	–
Cellular immunity	+	–	–	+
Immune regulation	+	–	+	+
Phagocytosis	–	–	–	+
Cytotoxicity	+	–	+	+
Receptor	TcR	IgM & IgD	CD16	CD11b
Other surface markers	CD3, CD4, CD8	CD19–21	CD56	CD14
Mononuclear cells in blood (%)	~75	~10	10	5

Table 2.
Major features and functions of mononuclear leukocytes.

DOI: http://dx.doi.org/10.5772/intechopen.81568

main receptors in the immune system are pattern recognition receptors (PRRs), Toll-like receptors (TLRs), killer activated and killer inhibitor receptors (KARs and KIRs), complement receptors, Fc receptors, and B & T cell receptors. Many are

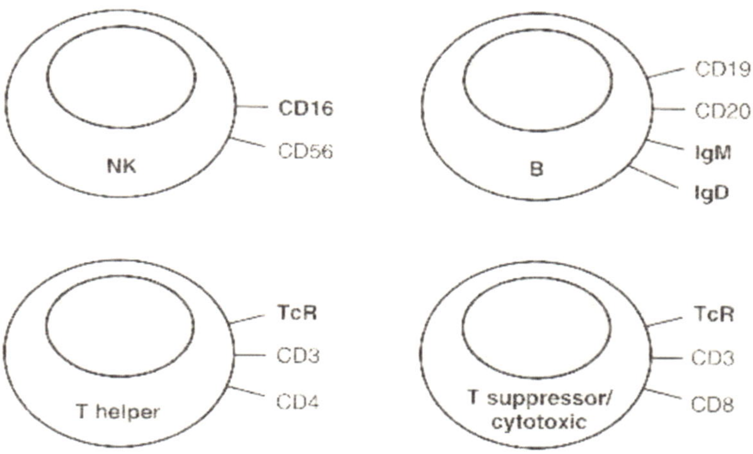

Figure 1.
Principal surface markers of lymphocyte populations.

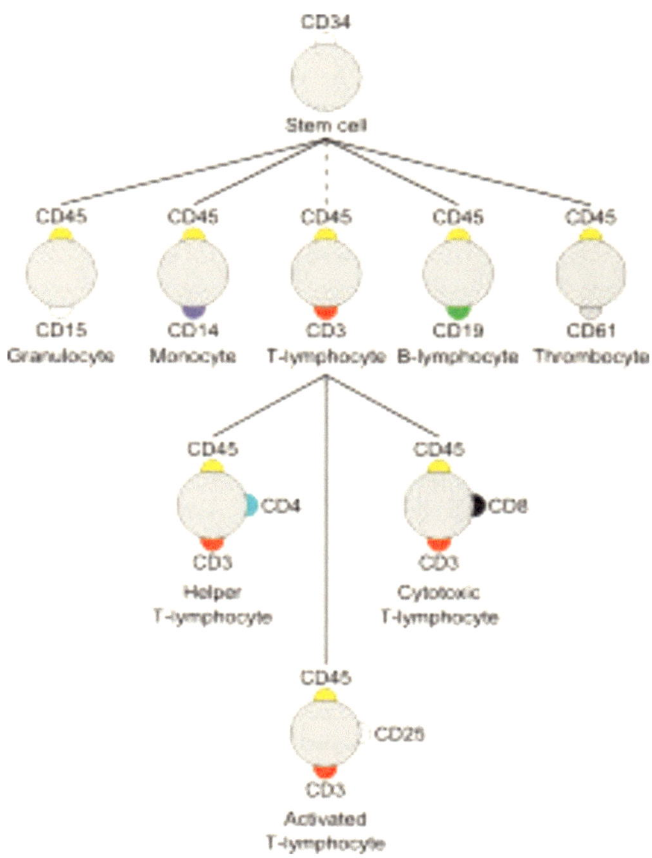

Figure 2.
Diagram showing CD markers on various immune cell types.

phagocytic receptors that stimulate ingestion of the pathogens they recognize. Some are chemotactic receptors, such as the f-Met-Leu-Phe receptor, which binds the N-formylated peptides produced by bacteria and guide neutrophils to sites of infection. A third function, which may be mediated by some of the phagocytic receptors as well as by specialized signaling receptors, is to induce effector molecules that contribute to induce innate immune responses and molecules that influence the initiation and nature of any subsequent adaptive immune response [1]. Various immune cell functions regulated by receptors on immunocytes are summarized in **Table 3** and **Figure 3**.

5. CD14 receptor coactivation with μOR: effect on cell division and NF-κB phosphorylation

LPS-mediated lymphocyte activation and effect of costimulation with opioid receptor agonists were studied by treating the cells with the μOR agonist DAMGO for time intervals of 5, 30, or 240 min. A549, a cell line having both CD14 and μOR, was used to study the effect on cell proliferation and NFκB phosphorylation. Treatment of A549 revealed that DAMGO was able to mitigate the LPS-mediated induction of phosphorylated NFκB after cotreatment for 4 h (**Figure 2**). Similarly, DAMGO was also able to suppress the cell proliferation by LPS, significantly reducing the percentage of cells in M-phase as well as in S-phase of the cell cycle (**Tables 2** and **3**).

Treatment	Cell population in M phase (%)	Paired T-test	Cell population in S-phase (%)	Paired T-test
LPS	6.07[1,2]		15.7[4, 5]	
DAMGO	4.83[1,3]	$P < 0.0001$[1]	10.5[4, 6]	$p = 0.029$[4]
LPS + DAMGO	3.89[2,3]	$P < 0.0001$[2], $p = 0.0018$[3]	7.99[5, 6]	$p = 0.0001$[5], $p = 0.002$[6]

[1]*NT vs. LPS.*
[2]*NT vs. DAMGO.*
[3]*NT vs. LPS + DAMGO.*
[4]*LPS vs. DAMGO.*
[5]*LPS vs. LPS + DAMGO.*
[6]*DAMGO vs. LPS + DAMGO.*

Table 3.
Effect of LPS and DAMGO on cell proliferation at 2 h after treatment.

6. Effect of μOR activation with a selective KOR agonist and μOR antagonist

The effect of coactivation of two different opioid receptors, U50488, a selective KOR agonist was used for lymphocyte activation, and effect of costimulation of μOR was achieved by using DAMGO, an opioid receptor agonist. Cells were treated with μOR agonists DAMGO for varying time intervals, and effect on cell proliferation and NF-κB phosphorylation was studied. Results using HepG2 revealed that U50488 (an agonist for KOR) was able to mitigate the effect of DAMGO, an agonist for μOR, and a significant reduction in the percentage of cells in both M-phase and S-phase of the cell cycle was observed at 2 and 24 h of treatment. U50488 alone also showed a larger percentage of cells in G0 phase both at 2 and 24 h in comparison with DAMGO, and the mitigation of U50488 induced effects indicating cross talk of receptors (**Figure 3**).

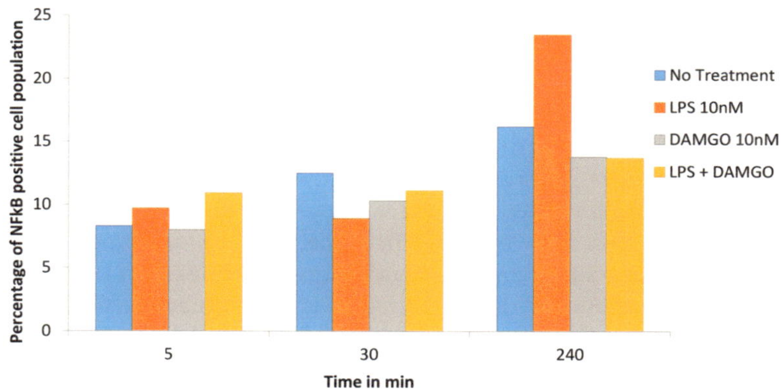

Figure 3.
Effect of cotreatment with agonist of OPRM1 (DAMGO) and agonist of CD-14 receptor (LPS) on NF-κB phosphorylation.

Treatment	Cell population in M phase (%)	Paired T-test	Cell population in S phase (%)	Paired T-test
DAMGO	26.66[1,2]		9.40[4,5]	
U50488	14.15[1,3]	$P < 0.0001$[1]	14.15[4,6]	$p < 0.001$[4]
U50488+ DAMGO	17.86[2,3]	$P < 0.0001$[2], $p < 0.0001$	8.07[5,6]	$p < 0.0001$[5] $p = 0.0002$[6]

1.[4]*DAMGO vs U50488.*
2.[5]*DAMGO vs U50488 + DAMGO.*
3.[6]*U50488 vs U50488+ DAMGO.*

Table 4.
Effect of U50488 and DAMGO on cell proliferation at 2 h after treatment.

Our studies show that U50488, agonist for κOR, was able to mitigate the effect of DAMGO, an agonist for MOR and a significant reduction in the percentage of cells in both M-phase and S-phase of cell cycle was observed at 2 and 24 h of treatment (**Table 4**).

7. Effect of μOR coactivation on cell proliferation

Receptor-receptor interactions and di/oligomerization are established pathways for altering response to any given ligand. As both homo- and heterodimers of μOR have been reported, it is speculated that dimerization of μOR may have a role in regulating receptor signaling. This intermolecular cross talk within receptor oligomers often results in allosterism between the different binding pockets of the individual monomers. Negative binding cooperativity has been observed for both GPCR homo- and heteromers using equilibrium binding and/or radio ligand dissociation [90].

Assays with TLR and μOR coactivation showed that agonist activation of μOR using DAMGO causes a significant lowering of LPS-induced cell division in cells coexpressing μOR and TLR. This has direct bearing on pathogen clearance as TLRs are present and expressed in sentinel cells such as macrophages and dendritic cells, which recognize structurally conserved molecules derived from microbes. These large phagocytes are found in essentially all tissues where they patrol for potential pathogens by amoeboid movement. These cells play a critical role in nonspecific defense (innate immunity) and also help initiate specific defense mechanisms (adaptive immunity) by recruiting other immune cells such as lymphocytes. Where a pathogen is involved, monocytes are commonly preceded by neutrophils, which release a range of toxic agents designed to kill extracellular pathogens. The macrophages then clear out both the dead pathogens and the dead neutrophils. The process of recruitment of neutrophils and macrophages involves the activation of resident macrophages. Activated resident macrophages respond to local stimuli by producing cytokines that make the endothelial cell surface more sticky (through induction of increased expression of cell adhesion molecules such as P-selectin) and chemokines, that promote and direct migration of inflammatory cells. Macrophages treated with LPS express high levels of cyclin D2 [91]. The CD14 and TLR signaling funnels into the activation of NF-κB, AP-1 and IRF3 pathways via the ERK1/2 and MEK1/2 channel, which is also activated by μOR signaling. Both signaling pathways funnel into the MAPK cascade and hence effect the activation of NFκB. Preliminary data from our study using both A549 and HepG2 cells show a significant decrease in LPS-induced cell division in the simultaneous presence of ligands for μOR. Cell cycle arrest was observed primarily in the S and the M phase of cell cycle with a significant decrease under conditions of costimulation with both the receptor agonists. Cell cycle arrest observed as a result of receptor coactivation needs to be further explored as it can have important therapeutic implications as on one hand a particular signaling pathway or end point is associated with a therapeutic response, such as analgesic effect of opioids, while on the other hand it is associated with unwanted side effects, namely cell cycle suppression on exposure to LPS and opioids together.

Receptor heteromers, with their allosteric properties, give rise to a new kind of pharmacological target. The ability of one of the protomers to act as an allosteric modulator of the second protomer in the receptor heteromer gives the possibility of finding selective ligands for the protomer acting as conduit of the allosteric modulation [73]. As opioid drugs are used in more than one clinical condition understanding opioid receptor interactions with other GPCRs on the surface of different cell types can prove to be very beneficial in managing adverse, unwanted effects of these important therapeutic molecules. The immunomodulatory effects of morphine have been characterized both in animal and human studies and was found to decrease several functions of both natural and acquired immunity, interfering with important intracellular pathways involved in immune regulation [92]. Opiates namely morphine, heroin, fentanyl and methadone all induce immune-suppression and affect both innate and adaptive immunity defining a role of μOR in these functions.

8. Association of OPRM1 functional alleles with immune cell function

Sharad et al. [93] used a genetic approach to correlate a functional *OPRM1* gene polymorphism with known action of opiates on immunity and undertook a prospective study to understand the relationship of the 118G variation with the amount of exogenous opiates consumed and correlated the immunosuppressive effects of exogenous opiates with the *OPRM1* allele type. They studied the immune status of opiate users by measuring serum Ig (IgG and IgA) levels, in association with specific *OPRM1* genotype, and confirmed that the mean circulating levels of Ig were significantly lower in opiate users when compared with levels in cohort controls. Among opiate-dependent subjects, individuals with AA genotype were found to have the lowest levels of circulating immunoglobulins, both IgG and IgA ($p = 0.0001$), while the AG genotype carrying individuals had a higher level of both immunoglobulins. The homozygous GG genotype was in between the AA and AG genotypes. Alternatively, in opiate naïve subjects, the AA individuals showed the highest titers of circulating IgG, and the GG individuals showed the lowest with AG having intermediate values [94]. The immunosuppressive effects documented in opiate naïve individuals can be attributed to altered regulation of PKA and pERK1/2 due to the levels of endogenous opioid. In addition to the absence of G genotype in the immortalized cell lines and based on the cell culture data showing cell cycle arrest observed in the present study (in A549 and HepG2 cell lines), we hypothesize that coactivation of μOR in presence of 118G allele leads to a suppression/arrest of cell division.

To test this hypothesis, another pilot study was carried out in which healthy opiate naïve volunteers were enrolled and the cell count for circulating lymphocyte subsets was studied as a measure of immune competence. Genotypic association studies showed a correlation between the immune cell numbers. Total lymphocyte count showed a significant lowering in cell numbers in 118G-allele-bearing individuals when compared to 118A-bearing individuals. However, cell numbers in all individuals remained within the documented normal range of 500–4000 cell/ml. The GG allele individuals showed significantly lower cell count, averaging 490, which differed markedly from cell numbers observed in AA-bearing individuals with mean numbers of 1976 cells/ml, ($p = 0.008$) and a correlation factor, r^2 of 0.79 between the genotype and average cell numbers. Our data show a significant lowering in all immunocytes, namely leucocyte populations (CD45+ve cells), B lymphocytes (CD10+ve cells), T lymphocytes (CD3, CD4, and CD8+ve cells), NK cells (CD56+ve cells), activated monocytes (CD 11b+ve cells), and mesenchymal progenitors in GG-bearing individuals when compared to AA-allele-bearing individuals but not always in comparison with those bearing the AG allele. This baseline lowering of cell numbers in GG-bearing individuals supports the hypothesis that GG genotype suppresses cell division, and since mounting of a successful immune response and/or overstimulation of immune system, as in case of patients with autoimmune disorders, depends on activation of both innate and adaptive immune responses, the 118G-bearing individuals would be prone to immune suppression due to lack of amplification by selective cell division, a critical step in elimination of the pathogen or an autoimmune response to an antigen.

9. Conclusion and future perspectives

In conclusion, there is a significant correlation between the circulating number of lymphocytes T_H and Tc, B cells and NK cells, and the μOR allele present, and this difference can be further increased in the presence of exogenous opioids either during clinical treatment or substance dependence, as the 118G allele affects the process of cell division arresting cells at the S or M phase of the cell cycle, or by modulating the action of cell division–linked secretion of stimulating cytokines/chemokine known to induce clone-specific and cell type–specific proliferation, because of the propensity of opioid receptor to heterodimerize and to selectively bias the subsequent ligand engagement/s with the dimerized/oligomerized receptors. This "subliminal immune suppression" in G allele–bearing individuals can have far reaching impact on onset of diseases such as cancer and obesity (both have an element inflammation) and vaccination for infectious diseases and even dreaded diseases as cancer. This immune suppression will certainly lower the individual's risk for autoimmune disorders such as rheumatoid arthritis, lupus, etc. The relationship between the μOR-mediated cell signaling and impact of stimulation of MOR as partner receptors, which influences binding of the second ligand in immunocytes and thereby the outcome on immune cells function in mounting and regulating the immune response/s, needs more detailed molecular exploration.

Author details

Suman Kapur* and Anuradha Pal
Birla Institute of Technology and Science (BITS Pilani), Hyderabad Campus, Hyderabad, Telangana, India

*Address all correspondence to: skapur@hyderabad.bits-pilani.ac.in

References

[1] Janeway CA Jr, Travers P, Walport M, et al. Receptors of the innate immune system. In: Immuno-biology: The Immune System in Health and Disease. 5th ed. New York: Garland Science; 2001. Available from: http://www.ncbi.nlm.nih.gov/books /NBK27129/

[2] Cooper MD, Peterson RD, Good RA. Delineation of the thymic and bursal lymphoid systems in the chicken. Nature. 1965;**205**:143-146

[3] Alberts B, Johnson A, Lewis J, et al. Chapter 24: The adaptive immune system. In: Molecular Biology of the Cell. 4th ed. New York: Garland Science; 2002. Available from: http://www.ncbi.nlm.nih.gov/books/NBK21070/

[4] Janković BD, Marić D. Enkephalins and immunity. I: In vivo suppression and potentiation of humoral immune response. Annals of the New York Academy of Sciences. 1987;**496**:115-125

[5] Wang J, Roderick Barke A, Sabita R. Transcriptional and epigenetic regulation of interleukin-2 Gene in activated T cells by morphine. The Journal of Biological Chemistry. 2007;**282**:7164-7171

[6] Vaswani M, Desai NG. HIV infection and high-risk behaviors in opioid dependent patients: The Indian context. Addictive Behaviors. 2004;**29**(8):1699-1705

[7] Sabita R, Jana N, Santanu B, Richard C, Subhas D, Raini D, et al. Opioid drug abuse and modulation of immune function: Consequences in the susceptibility to opportunistic infections. Journal of NeuroImmune Pharmacology. 2011;**6**(4):442-465

[8] Chang SL, Moldow RL, House SD, Zadina JE. Morphine affects the brain-immune axis by modulating an interleukin-1 beta dependent pathway. Advances in Experimental Medicine and Biology. 1996;**402**:35-42

[9] Bryant HU, Bernton EW, Holaday JW. Immunosuppressive effects of chronic morphine treatment in mice. Life Sciences. 1987;**41**(14):1731-1738

[10] Lefkowitz SS, Chiang CY. Effects of certain abused drugs on hemolysin forming cells. Life Sciences. 1975;**17**(12):1763-1767

[11] Güngör M et al. Effect of chronic administration of morphine on primary immune response in mice. Experientia. 1980;**36**(11):1309-1310

[12] Tubaro E, Borelli G, Croce C, Cavallo G, Santiangeli C. Effect of morphine on resistance to infection. The Journal of Infectious Diseases. 1983;**148**(4):656-666

[13] Chao CC, Sharp BM, Pomeroy C, Filice GA, Peterson PK. Lethality of morphine in mice infected with *Toxoplasma gondii*. The Journal of Pharmacology and Experimental Therapeutics. 1990;**252**(2):605-609

[14] Fecho K, Manning EL, Maixner W, Schmitt CP. Effects of carrageenan and morphine on acute inflammation and pain in Lewis and Fischer rats. Brain, Behavior, and Immunity. 2007;**21**(1):68-78

[15] Novick DM, Ochshorn M, Ghali V, Croxson TS, Mercer WD, Chiorazzi N, et al. Natural killer cell activity and lymphocyte subsets in parenteral heroin abusers and long-term methadone maintenance patients. The Journal of Pharmacology and Experimental Therapeutics. 1989;**250**(2):606-610

[16] Taub DD, Eisenstein TK, Geller EB, Adler MW, Rogers TJ. Immunomodulatory activity of mu- and kappa-selective opioid agonists. Proceedings of the National

Academy of Sciences of the United States of America. 1991;**88**(2):360-364

[17] Roy JD, Massicotte L, Sassine MP, Seal RF, Roy A. A comparison of intrathecal morphine/fentanyl and patient-controlled analgesia with patient-controlled analgesia alone for analgesia after liver resection. Anesthesia and Analgesia. 2006;**103**(4):990-994

[18] Carr DJ, Kim CH, de Costa B, Jacobson AE, Rice KC, Blalock JE. Evidence for a delta-class opioid receptor on cells of the immune system. Cellular Immunology. 1988;**116**(1):44-51

[19] Carr DJ, DeCosta BR, Kim CH, Jacobson AE, Guarcello V, Rice KC, et al. Opioid receptors on cells of the immune system: Evidence for delta- and kappa-classes. The Journal of Endocrinology. 1989;**122**(1):161-168

[20] Chuang TK, Killam KF, Chuang LF, Kung HF, Sheng WS, Chao CC, et al. Mu opioid receptor gene expression in immune cells. Biochemical and Biophysical Research Communications. 1995;**216**(3):922-930

[21] Chao CC, Gekker G, Hu S, Sheng WS, Shark KB, Bu DF, et al. Kappa opioid receptors in human microglia downregulate human immunodeficiency virus 1 expression. Proceedings of the National Academy of Sciences of the United States of America. 1996;**93**(15):8051-8056

[22] Royal W 3rd, Leander MV, Bissonnette R. Retinoid-induced mu opioid receptor expression by phyto-hemagglutinin-stimulated U937 cells. Journal of Neurovirology. 2005;**11**(2):157-165

[23] Wetzel MA, Steele AD, Eisenstein TK, Adler MW, Henderson EE, Rogers TJ. μ-Opioid induction of monocyte chemoattractant protein-1, RANTES, and IFN-γ-inducible protein-10 expression in human peripheral blood mononuclear cells. The Journal of Immunology. 2000;**165**(11):6519-6524

[24] Simpkins CO, Dickey CA, Fink MP. Human neutrophil migration is enhanced by beta-endorphin. Life Sciences. 1984;**34**(23):2251-2255

[25] Van Epps DE, Saland L. Beta-endorphin and met-enkephalin stimulate human peripheral blood mononuclear cell chemotaxis. Journal of Immunology. 1984;**132**(6):3046-3053

[26] Grimm MC, Ben-Baruch A, Taub DD, Howard OMZ, Resau JH, Wang JM, et al. Opiates Trans-deactivate Chemokine Receptors: δ and μ Opiate Receptor–mediated Heterologous Desensitization. The Journal of Experimental Medicine. 1998;**188**(2):317-325

[27] Liu Y, Blackbourn DJ, Chuang LF, Killam KF Jr, Chuang RY. Effects of in vivo and in vitro administration of morphine sulfate upon rhesus macaque polymorphonuclear cell phagocytosis and chemotaxis. The Journal of Pharmacology and Experimental Therapeutics. 1992;**263**(2):533-539

[28] Ruff MR, Wahl SM, Mergenhagen S, Pert CB. Opiate receptor-mediated chemotaxis of human monocytes. Neuropeptides. 1985;**5**(4-6):363-366

[29] Makman MH, Dvorkin B, Stefano G. Murine macrophage cell lines contain mu 3-opiate receptors. European Journal of Pharmacology. 1995;**273**(3):R5-R6

[30] Bowdle TA. Adverse effects of opioid agonists and agonists-antagonists in anesthesia. Drug Safety. 1998;**19**:173-189

[31] Brown SM, Stimmel B, Taub RN, Kochwa S, Rosenfield RE. Immunologic dysfunction in heroin addicts. Archives of Internal Medicine. 1974;**134**(6):1001-1006

[32] Noel RJ. Opiates, immune system, acquired immunodeficiency syndrome, and nonhuman primate model. Journal of Neurovirology. 2008;**4**:279-285

[33] Miyagi AU et al. Opioids suppress chemokine-mediated migration of monkey neutrophils and monocytes—An instant response. Immunopharmacology. 2000;**47**:53-62

[34] Perez-Castrillon JL, Pérez-Arellano JL, García-Palomo JD, Jiménez-López A, De Castro SL. Opioids depress in vitro human monocyte chemotaxis. Immunopharmacology. 1992;**23**(1):57-61

[35] Donahoe RM. Neuro-immuno-modulation by opiates: Relationship to HIV infection and AIDS. Advances in Neuroimmunology. 1993;**3**:31-46

[36] McDonough RJ, Madden JJ, Falek A, Shafer DA, Pline M, Gordon D, et al. Alteration of T and null lymphocyte frequencies in the peripheral blood of human opiate addicts: In vivo evidence for opiate receptor sites on T lymphocytes. Journal of Immunology. 1980;**125**(6):2539-2543

[37] DesJarlais DC, Friedman SR, Marmor M. Development of AIDS, HIV seroconversion, and potential cofactors for T4 cell loss in a cohort of I.V. drug users. AIDS. 1987;**1**:105-111

[38] Culver KW, Ammann AJ, Partridge JC, Wong DF, Wara DW, Cowan MJ. Lymphocyte abnormalities in infants born to drug-abusing mothers. The Journal of Pediatrics. 1987;**111**(2):230-235

[39] Mientjers GH, Miedema F, van Ameijden EJ, van den Hoek AA, Schellekens PT, Roos MT, et al. Frequent injecting impairs lymphocyte reactivity in HIV-positive and HIV-negative drug users. AIDS. 1991;**5**(1):35-41

[40] Rouveix B. Opiates and immune function: Consequences on infectious diseases with special reference to AIDS. Thérapie. 1992;**47**:503-512

[41] Thomas PT, Bhargava HN, House RV. Immunomodulatory effects of in vitro exposure to morphine and its metabolites. Pharmacology. 1995;**50**(1):51-62

[42] Varela P, Marcos A, Santacruz I, Ripoll S, Requejo AM. Human immunodeficiency virus infection and nutritional status in female drug addicts undergoing detoxification: Anthropometric and immunologic assessments. The American Journal of Clinical Nutrition. 1997;**66**(2):504S-508S

[43] Rho YM. Infections as fatal complications of narcotism. New York State Journal of Medicine. 1972;**72**:823-830

[44] Islam M, Frye RF, Richards TJ, Sbeitan I, Donnelly SS, Glue P, et al. Differential effect of IFNalpha-2b on the cytochrome P450 enzyme system: A potential basis of IFN toxicity and its modulation by other drugs. Clinical Cancer Research. 2000;**8**(8):2480-2507

[45] Islam N, Kanost AR, Teixeira L, Johnson J, Hejal R, Aung H, et al. Role of cellular activation and tumor necrosis factor-alpha in the early expression of mycobacterium tuberculosis 85B mRNA in human alveolar macrophages. The Journal of Infectious Diseases. 2004;**190**(20):341-351

[46] Islam SK, Hossain KJ, Kamal M, Ahsan M. Serum immunoglobulins and white blood cells status of drug addicts: Influence of illicit drugs and sex habit. Addiction Biology. 2004;**9**(1):27-33

[47] Naik S, Vaswani M, Desai NG. Humoral immune function in non-parenteral heroin dependence: Indian data. Alcoholism. 2001;**37**(1):25-34

[48] Roudebush RE et al. Dissociation of immunosuppression by chlorpromazine and trifluoperazine from

pharmacologic activities as dopamine antagonists. International Journal of Immunopathology and Pharmacology. 1991;**13**(7):961-968

[49] Bidlack JM. Detection and function of opioid receptors on cells from the immune system. Clinical and Diagnostic Laboratory Immunology. 2000;**7**(5):719-723

[50] Hoehe MR, Köpke K, Wendel B, Rohde K, Flachmeier C, Kidd KK, et al. Sequence variability and candidate gene analysis in complex disease: Association of mu opioid receptor gene variation with substance dependence. Human Molecular Genetics. 2000;**9**:2895-2908

[51] Margas W, Zubkoff I, Schuler HG, Janicki PK, Ruiz-Velasco V. Modulation of Ca^{2+} channels by heterologously expressed wild-type and mutant human micro-opioid receptors (hMORs) containing the A118G single nucleotide polymorphism. Journal of Neurophysiology. 2007;**97**(2):1058-1067

[52] Kroslak T, Laforge KS, Gianotti RJ, Ho A, Nielsen DA, Kreek MJ. The single nucleotide polymorphism A118G alters functional properties of the human mu opioid receptor. Journal of Neurochemistry. 2007;**103**(1):77-87

[53] Deb I, Chakraborty J, Gangopadhyay PK, Choudhury SR, Das S. Single-nucleotide polymorphism (A118G) in exon 1 of OPRM1 gene causes alteration in downstream signaling by mu-opioid receptor and may contribute to the genetic risk for addiction. Journal of Neurochemistry. 2010;**112**(2):486-496

[54] Zhang Y, Wang D, Johnson AD, Papp AC, Sadée W. Allelic expression imbalance of human mu opioid receptor (OPRM1) caused by variant A118G. The Journal of Biological Chemistry. 2005;**280**:32618-32624

[55] Pang GS, Wang J, Wang Z, Goh C, Lee CG. The G allele of SNP E1/A118G at the mu-opioid receptor gene locus shows genomic evidence of recent positive selection. Pharmacogenomics. 2009;**10**(7):1101-1109

[56] Huang P, Chen C, Mague SD, Blendy JA, Liu-Chen LY. A common single nucleotide polymorphism A118G of the μ-opioid receptor alters its N-glycosylation and protein stability. The Biochemical Journal. 2012;**441**(1):379-386

[57] Garden Gardiner and Frommer M&M. CpG islands in vertebrate genomes. Journal of Molecular Biology. 1987;**196**:261-282

[58] Nielsen DA, Vadim Y, Sara H, Colin J, Ann H, Jurg O, et al. Increased OPRM1 DNA methylation in lymphocytes of methadone-maintained former heroin addicts. Neuropsychopharmacology. 2009;**34**:867-873

[59] Chorbov VM, Todorov AA, Lynskey MT, Cicero TJ. Elevated levels of DNA methylation at the OPRM1 promoter in blood and sperm from male opioid addicts. Journal of Opioid Management. 2011;7(4):258-264

[60] Oertel BG, Doehring A, Roskam B, et al. Genetic-epigenetic interaction modulates μ-opioid receptor regulation. Human Molecular Genetics. 2012;**21**(21):4751-4760

[61] Johnson AD, Zhang Y, Papp AC, et al. Polymorphisms affecting gene transcription and mRNA processing in pharmacogenetic candidate genes: Detection through allelic expression imbalance in human target tissues. Pharmacogenetics and Genomics. 2008;**18**(9):781-791

[62] Goddard Alan D, Anthony W. Regulation of G protein-coupled receptors by palmitoylation and cholesterol. BMC Biology. 2012;**10**:27

[63] Maurice P, Kamal M, Jockers R. Asymmetry of GPCR oligomers supports their functional relevance.

Trends in Pharmacological Sciences. 2011;**32**(9):514-520

[64] Krzysztof P. Oligomeric forms of G protein-coupled receptors (GPCRs). Trends in Biochemical Sciences. 2010;**35**(11):595-600

[65] Park PS, Filipek S, Wells JW, Palczewski K. Oligomerization of G protein-coupled receptors: Past, present, and future. Biochemistry. 2004;**43**(50):15643-15656

[66] Mansoor SE, Palczewski K, Farrens DL. Rhodopsin self-associates in asolectin liposomes. Proceedings of the National Academy of Sciences of the United States of America. 2006;**103**(9):3060-3065

[67] Rovira X, Pin JP, Giraldo J. The asymmetric/symmetric activation of GPCR dimers as a possible mechanistic rationale for multiple signaling pathways. Trends in Pharmacological Sciences. 2010;**31**(1):15-21

[68] Arcemisbéhère L, Sen T, Boudier L, Balestre M-N, Gaibelet G, Detouillon E, et al. Leukotriene BLT2 receptor monomers activate the G (i2) GTP-binding protein more efficiently than dimers. The Journal of Biological Chemistry. 2010;**285**:6337-6347

[69] Milligan G. G protein-coupled receptor hetero-dimerization: Contribution to pharmacology and function. British Journal of Pharmacology. 2009;**158**(1):5-14

[70] Maggio R, Aloisi G, Silvano E, Rossi M, Millan MJ. Heterodimerization of dopamine receptors: New insights into functional and therapeutic significance. Parkinsonism & Related Disorders. 2009;**15**(S4):S2-S7

[71] Vischer HF, Nijmeijer S, Smit MJ, Leurs R. Viral hijacking of human receptors through heterodimerization. Biochemical and Biophysical Research Communications. 2008;**377**(1):93-97

[72] Zhang M, Feng X, Guan R, Hébert TE, Segaloff DL. A cell surface inactive mutant of the human lutropin receptor (hLHR) attenuates signaling of wild-type or constitutively active receptors via heterodimerization. Cellular Signalling. 2009;**21**(11):1663-1671

[73] Sergi F, Vicent C, Devi LA, Marta F, Ralf J, Lohse MJ, et al. G protein–coupled receptor oligomerization revisited: Functional and pharmacological perspectives. Pharmacological Reviews. 2014;**66**(2):413-434

[74] Golebiewska U, Johnston JM, Devi L, Filizola M, Scarlata S. Differential response to morphine of the oligomeric state of μ-opioid in the presence of δ-opioid receptors. Biochemistry. 2011;**50**(14):2829-2837

[75] Manglik A, Kruse AC, Kobilka TS, Thian FS, Mathiesen JM, Sunahara RK, et al. Crystal structure of the μ-opioid receptor bound to a morphine antagonist. Nature. 2012;**485**(7398):321-326

[76] Huang J, Chen S, Zhang JJ, Huang XY. Crystal structure of oligomeric β1-adrenergic G protein-coupled receptors in ligand-free basal state. Nature Structural & Molecular Biology. 2013;**20**(4):419-425

[77] Gomes I, Gupta A, Filipovska J, Szeto HH, Pintar JE, Devi LA. A role for heterodimerization of mu and delta opiate receptors in enhancing morphine analgesia. Proceedings of the National Academy of Sciences of the United States of America. 2004;**101**(14):5135-5139

[78] Gomes I, Ijzerman AP, Ye K, Maillet EL, Devi LA. G protein-coupled receptor heteromerization: A role in allosteric modulation of ligand binding. Molecular Pharmacology. 2011;**79**(6):1044-1052

[79] Bushlin I, Gupta A, Stockton SD Jr, Miller LK, Devi LA. Dimerization with

cannabinoid receptors allosterically modulates delta opioid receptor activity during neuropathic pain. PLoS One. 2012;**7**(12):e49789

[80] Rozenfeld R, Bushlin I, Gomes I, Tzavaras N, Gupta A, Neves S, et al. Receptor heteromerization expands the repertoire of cannabinoid signaling in rodent neurons. PLoS One. 2012;**7**(1):e29239

[81] Gupta A, Mulder J, Gomes I, Rozenfeld R, Bushlin I, Ong E, et al. Increased abundance of opioid receptor heteromers after chronic morphine administration. Science Signaling. 2010;**3**(131):ra54

[82] Zheng H, Pearsall EA, Hurst DP, Zhang Y, Chu J, Zhou Y, et al. Palmitoylation and membrane cholesterol stabilize μ-opioid receptor homodimerization and G protein coupling. BMC Cell Biology. 2012;**13**:6

[83] Zhang N, Oppenheim JJ. Crosstalk between chemokines and neuronal receptors bridges immune and nervous systems. Journal of Leukocyte Biology. 2005;**78**(6):1210-1214

[84] Murphy PM. Chemokine receptors: Structure, function and role in microbial pathogenesis. Cytokine & Growth Factor Reviews. 1996;**7**(1):47-64

[85] Snyderman R, Uhing RJ. Chemoattractant stimulus-response coupling. In: Gallin JI, Goldstein IM, Snyderman R, editors. Inflammation: Basic Principles and Clinical Correlates. 2nd ed. New York: Raven Press, Ltd.; 1992. pp. 421-439

[86] Ali H, Tomhave ED, Richardson RM, Haribabu B, Snyderman R. Thrombin primes responsiveness of selective chemoattractant receptors at a site distal to G protein activation. The Journal of Biological Chemistry. 1996;**271**(6):3200-3206

[87] Ben-Baruch A, Grimm M, Bengali K, Evans GA, Chertov O, Wang JM, et al. The differential ability of IL-8 and neutrophil-activating peptide-2 to induce attenuation of chemotaxis is mediated by their divergent capabilities to phosphorylate CXCR2 (IL-8 receptor B). Journal of Immunology. 1997;**158**(12):5927-5933

[88] Imre S, Xiao-Hong C, Li X, Adler MW, Howard OMZ, Oppenheim JJ, et al. Heterologous desensitization of opioid receptors by chemokines inhibits chemotaxis and enhances the perception of pain. Proceedings of the National Academy of Sciences of the United States of America. 2002;**99**(16):10276-10281

[89] Goldman AS, Prabhakar BS. Chapter 1: Immunology overview. In: Baron S, editor. Medical Microbiology. 4th ed. Galveston, TX: University of Texas Medical Branch at Galveston; 1996. http://www.ncbi.nlm.nih.gov/books/NBK7795/

[90] Springa JY, Urizar E, Costagliola S, Vassart G, Parmentier M. Allosteric properties of G protein-coupled receptor oligomers. Pharmacology & Therapeutics. 2007;**115**(3):410-418

[91] Vadiveloo PK. Macrophages—Proliferation, activation, and cell cycle proteins. Journal of Leukocyte Biology. 1999;**66**(4):579-582

[92] Sacerdote P. Opioid-induced immunosuppression. Current Opinion in Supportive and Palliative Care. 2008;**2**(1):14-18

[93] Sharad S, Gupta AK, Singh RA, Kapoor M, Kapur S. Correlation of circulatory immunoglobulin levels with mu opiate receptor allele. Indian Journal of Biochemistry & Biophysics. 2007;**44**(5):394-400

[94] Kapur S, Pal A, Sharad S. Role of Opioidergic System in Humoral Immune Response. Immunosuppression—Role in Health and Diseases. Rijeka, Croatia: InTech; 2012

Section 3

Immunomodulation

Chapter 6

Mesenchymal Stem Cells Modulate the Immune System in Developing Therapeutic Interventions

Sonali Rawat, Suchi Gupta and Sujata Mohanty

Abstract

Mesenchymal stem cells (MSCs) are emerging as key players in regenerative medicine for the treatment of various diseases associated with the inflammation and degeneration, thereby aiding in therapeutic advancements. Several tissues have been identified as potential sources of MSCs including the bone marrow, cord blood, dental pulp, umbilical cord, adipose tissue, peripheral blood, and fetal liver, of which some are clinically recognized. MSCs are capable of differentiating into cells of multiple lineages and therefore established as suitable candidates for transplantation in damaged organs. They have added advantage of higher proliferation, easy expansion, and, more importantly, the absence of HLA class II receptors, with potential applications extending toward allogenic settings. MSCs are actively involved in different mechanisms related to repair and regeneration of tissues via immunomodulation, transdifferentiation, paracrine factors, etc. They are known to exhibit profound immunomodulatory effect on T and B cells and natural killer (NK) cells mediated via soluble factors and direct cell-cell contact. The MSCs activate the immune responses and inhibit proliferation, maturation, and differentiation of T and B cells. The MSC-activated immune responses induce the expression of regulatory T cells (Tregs). A plethora of studies have established that MSCs suppress immune responses via immunomodulation that makes them a preferred cell source for the use in clinical trials.

Keywords: MSCs, therapeutic, immunomodulatory, GvHD

1. Introduction

Stem cells are undifferentiated cells possessing greater capacity of self-renewal and multilineage differentiation potential. This makes them unique candidates for curing a diverse variety of human degenerative diseases. Based on their potency, stem cells are classified into three broad groups: embryonic stem cells (ESCs), fetal stem cells (FSCs), and adult stem cells (ASC). ESCs are pluripotent stem cells isolated from inner cell mass of blastocysts of human embryos. The uniqueness of ESCs lies in the fact that they are capable of differentiation into all three primary germ layers, i.e., ectoderm, endoderm, and mesoderm. However, due to high tendency of teratoma formation and ethical issues regarding the destruction of human embryos, the clinical applications of ESCs are restricted. Alternatively, fetal and adult tissue-derived stem cells are gaining popularity with little ethical concerns. Fetal stem cells can be isolated from extraembryonic tissues like cord blood, amniotic fluid, Wharton's jelly, the placenta, and amniotic membrane [1–3]. However, adult stem cells (ASCs) are multipotent cells and are usually harvested from the bone marrow, adipose tissue, dental pulp, etc. All together, these cells possess clonogenic and self-renewing potential and plasticity to differentiate and often transdifferentiate into different tissue types.

Isolated stem cells from both adult and fetal tissues are multipotent and are recognized as MSCs. Notably, despite similar morphology and phenotypic properties, these tissue-specific MSCs have subtle differences in their regenerative potential due to the impact of stem cell niche on cell fate, known as stem cell niche theory, genetic variability, and/or epigenetic alterations [4]. Several studies have been carried out to show that there are differences in regenerative capacity of MSCs populations of

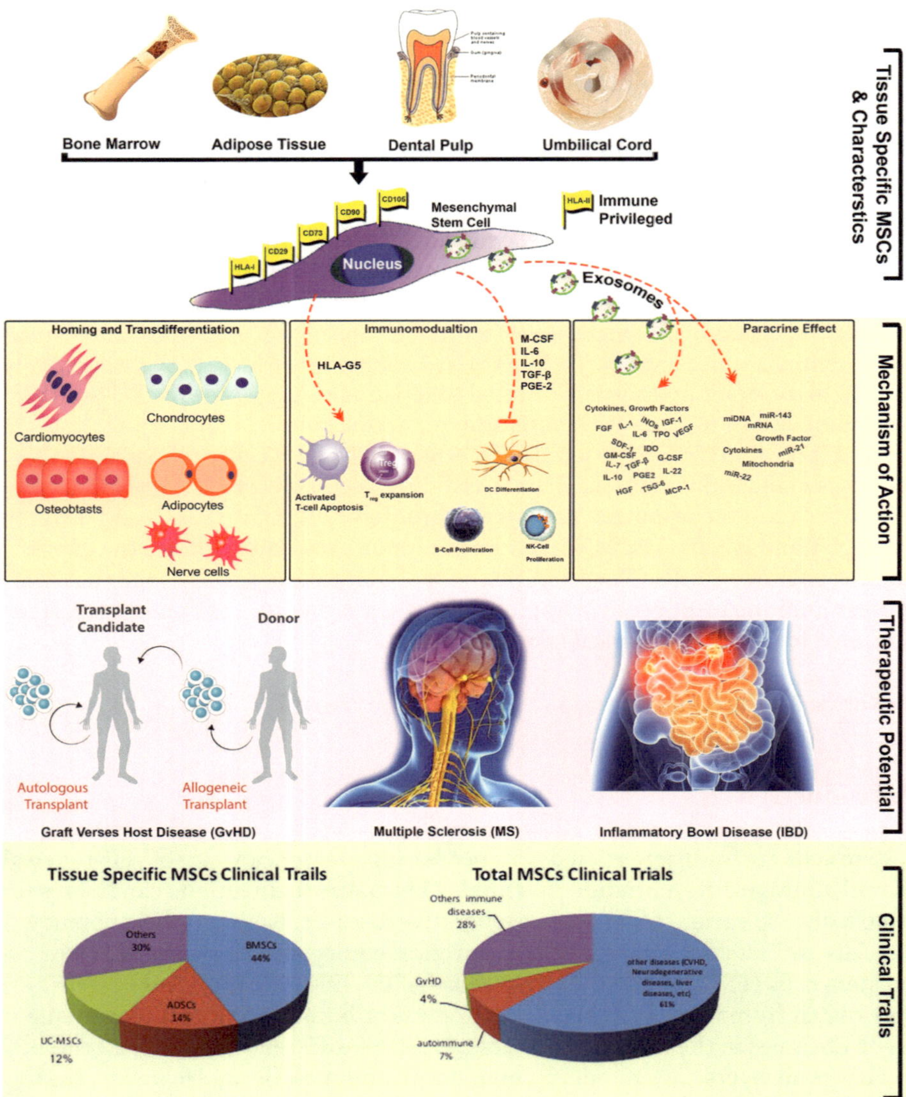

Figure 1.
A diagrammatic representation of cellular characteristics, mode of action, and their therapeutic potential of mesenchymal stem cells with current status of clinical trial.

the same passage number that have been isolated from different pockets of the body [5]. A recent comprehensive report also supports the hypothesis that tissue-specific MSCs express certain source-specific markers [6]. Dominic et al. established criteria to define MSCs on the basis of the following characteristics: (1) plastic-adherent cells; (2) expression of surface markers, CD73, CD90, CD105, and HLA-ABC, but negative expression from hematopoietic lineage-specific markers, CD34, CD45, CD14, CD11b, CD19, or HLA-DR; and (3) potential to differentiate into trilineage, i.e., osteoblast, adipocytes, and chondrocytes [7].

Due to their enhanced regenerative potential, the use of MSCs has become an emerging strategy for the treatment of injured or degenerated tissues. It was observed that in in vivo scenario, MSCs showed profound immunomodulatory effect [8]. The most important characteristic of MSCs is its immunomodulatory property which augments and modulates both adaptive and innate immune responses as it initiates the wound healing paradigm.

MSCs are also known for their immune-privileged property due to their low immunogenicity. Human MSCs show low levels of human leukocyte antigen (HLA) class I, and they do not express HLA-DR which is necessary to escape immune surveillance. The presence of HLA class I is important as low levels of HLA class I protect cells from the natural killer (NK) cell-mediated cytotoxicity. On the contrary, cells which do not express HLA class I are targeted and destroyed easily. Another essential characteristic is that they home and migrate to the site of damage where there is secretion of inflammatory chemokines. These events are mediated by several chemokine receptors which aid in their migration and homing potential to the sites of inflammation [9]. Owing to the immune tolerance property of MSCs, they possess several clinical advantages due to which these cells are also referred as "universal donors" [10, 11]. However, as true with any other cell-based therapy, the evaluation of safety and efficacy of these MSCs in allogeneic strategies for clinical use is of utmost importance (**Figure 1**).

The initial reports of immunoregulatory properties were started with bone marrow-derived MSCs (BM-MSCs) [12]. Later, other sources of MSCs such as adipose tissue-derived MSCs (AD-MSCs) and Wharton's jelly-derived MSCs (WJ-MSCs) were also explored for their immunomodulatory properties [1].

However, several challenges need to be overcome prior to the clinical applications of MSCs. Hence, a thorough insight of the various biological properties of MSCs will elucidate the mechanisms of MSC-based transplantation for immunomodulation.

2. Immunoregulatory function of MSCs in the inflammatory microenvironment

A key factor of survival in multicellular organisms is the maintenance and balance of homeostatic state. In the absence of inflammation, phagocytic cell is recruited to remove the apoptotic cells, whereas during acute injury, it is accompanied by inflammation, and the cell components that are released from necrotic cells result in microvascular damage due to increased vasopermeability and infiltration of macrophages and neutrophils [13]. During the process of phagocytosis of necrotic cells, there is secretion of pro-inflammatory mediators such as interleukin-1 (IL-1), interferon-γ (IFN-γ), and tumor necrosis factor-α (TNF-α), various chemokines which further initiate downstream signaling pathways [14]. Adaptive immune response actively participates in the repair of damaged tissues in close association with CD4+, CD8+, T, and B cells [13]. Recently, MSCs have been recognized to be actively involved in damaged tissue repair processes. As a functional unit for development and regeneration in various tissues, they hold utmost importance in maintaining proper functioning of tissues [15, 16]. In their undifferentiated and self-renewable state, the balance among interaction and protection of MSCs appears to be achieved by maintaining the stem cells in a specialized microenvironment called "niche." This niche provides accommodation to different molecules to brace and coordinate stem cell activities pertaining to growth, proliferation, differentiation, and functionality. In particular, cell-cell interaction in the niche provides structural support, regulates adhesive interaction, and activates signals by secretion of certain molecules that can control stem cell functions. Stem cell immunoregulatory responses occur due to its close association with vasculature which provides metabolic cues and a conduit due to which inflammatory cytokines and immune cells, as well as humoral factors, can be delivered to the niche. In addition, the niche also provides biochemical and biomechanical parameters such as temperature, shear force, and chemical signals, which also influence stem cell behavior and fate in response to the external environment. In the process of tissue repair, MSCs are able to affect the inflamed microenvironment by secreting a cascade of various adhesion molecules, growth factors, and pro- and anti-inflammatory cytokines [17]. Since MSCs display notable immunomodulatory properties and they are able to dodge the immune system recognition mechanisms, they can potentially modulate the defense mechanisms of the host. In inflammatory condition, MSCs located in immediate location or originating from the bone marrow region start migrating to the site of injury. At the site, these MSCs associate themselves closely with numerous types of immune cells in order to initiate regeneration process of damaged tissue, which is typically accompanied with cytokine storm. The combinational sensitization of MSCs by IFN-γ and TNF-α induces the release of chemokines where they participate in chemotaxis and are able to inhibit proliferation of inflammatory effector cells. Several molecules participate in the activation, homing, and functionality of MSCs [18] (**Figure 2**). The commencement of homing process is led by selectins present on the endothelium. Specifically, for bone marrow homing, the expression of hematopoietic cell E-/L-selectin ligand (HCELL) is very important which is a functional glycoform of CD44 present on the migrating cells, while MSCs do not express HCELL but express CD44. The subsequent molecules participated in the activation of MSCs are mainly chemokine receptors [19, 20].

Chemokines are defined as positively charged short peptides (7–13 kDa). Broadly, four families of chemokines have been recognized: CCL family with adjacent cysteine residues, CXCL family with cysteine residues separated by a single amino acid, CXCL family with two instead of four cysteines, and CX3CL family with cysteines separated by three amino acids. For MSCs to home to injury site, these cells bear chemokine receptors and are identified at site of injury due to production of the chemokines. Hence a thorough understanding of the functioning of chemokine receptor profile is important for optimizing the process of both internal and external homing processes of MSCs to wound site. The site of injury produces abundant chemokines which may provide signal to MSCs or may function as chemoattractants [21]. During the process of regeneration or repair, the injury site tightly regulates the process of chemokine expression profile or expression pattern of each chemokine, which plays a unique role in directed migration of cells toward the site of injury. The subsequent expression of chemokines to attract specific immune cell types is conducted by immune response of injury.

Integrins are key players associated with the balance activation-dependent arrest of MSCs in the second last step of homing. They are known for cell-cell mediated matrix and adhesion, and they belong to the largest family of receptors. Mammals contain 18α and 18β subunits of integrin that combine to form at least 24 different heterodimers, each of which corresponds to a specific set of cell surface,

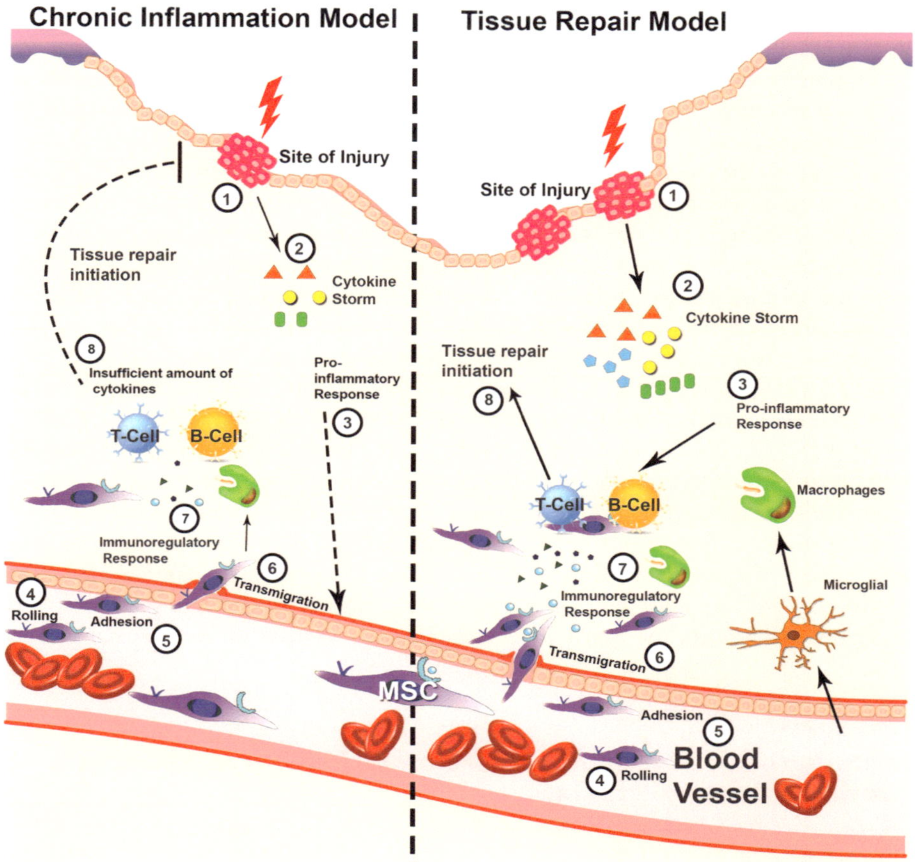

Figure 2.
Immunoregulatory action of MSCs at chronic inflammation (left panel) versus acute inflammation (right panel). MSCs home to the injury site due to local cytokine storm secreted by activated immune cells. Activation and migration of MSCs lead to secretion of multiple immunomodulatory and growth factors. Depending on the cytokine signal (acute versus chronic inflammation), MSCs initiate the immunoregulatory response and repair the injury site or are unable to inhibit the persisting chronic inflammatory signals resulting in cellular fibrosis.

extracellular matrix (ECM) or soluble protein ligands. They are multifaceted receptors, transmitting bidirectional signals across the cell membrane, which is crucial for building a suitable interaction between the exterior and interior of the cell. Numerous cell processes like morphology, migration, proliferation, differentiation, and apoptosis are unexpected on this recurrent discussion. According to few reports, it was suggested that MSC homing will be affected if integrin-β1 is inhibited. Also, interaction of vascular cell adhesion molecule-1-very late antigen-4 (VCAM1-VL4) is involved functionally in MSC homing [22].

During the last stage of transmigration across the endothelial cell layer and below the basement membrane, various lytic enzymes are essential to cleave components of the basement membrane, such as the matrix metalloproteinases (MMPs) [23]. Specifically, gelatinases, MMP-2 and MMP-9, preferentially degrade collagen and gelatin, two of the major components of the basement membrane which facilitate MSC migration. The MSCs reportedly help migrate MMP-2 and tissue inhibitor of metalloproteinases 3 (TIMP-3) [23].

The initial reports pointing to MSC homing were toward investigating the origin of BM-MSCs after allogeneic bone marrow transplantation. Those studies also concluded that the hematopoietic cell population was provided by the donor, but the stem cells were provided by the recipient [24]. Therefore, a number of trials at both the preclinical and clinical levels have been carried out, and MSCs are seen to help migrate in a variety of tissues. Initial studies in animal models also confirmed that the presence of MSCs transplanted to donor was present in the bone marrow, thymus, spleen, and liver [12, 24, 25].

To elucidate the dynamics of MSCs migration, a systemic infusion of MSCs was studied by using varied techniques, i.e., after infusion of MSCs, they were first trapped in the lungs, and eventually, the cells disappear from the lungs and are distributed to other organs. Other aspects of MSCs homing was also studied by few groups under which they studied the factors such as early cell passage, irradiation and younger animals and observed that they influence the short-term bone marrow homing and condition which in result increases the homing [26–30].

Once MSCs are activated and recruited to the site of injury, there is onset of T-cell activation because of the presence of various pro-inflammatory cytokines such as IFN-γ, TNF-α, IL-1β, etc. IFN-γ is a critical player in providing stimulatory signals for activation and expansion of T cells and its subsets, such as it begins to suppress the T cell proliferation, differentiation, and inhibition of various biological functions. Other than IFN-γ, TNF-α and IL-1β also activate MSCs, either in synergy or alone. After stimulation with pro-inflammatory cytokines, MSCs also release other significant immunomodulatory factors. These stimulated cells modulate many immune effecters in vitro as well as in an animal model [31, 32].

3. Secretion of anti-inflammatory factors by MSCs is regulated by pro-inflammatory cytokines

To participate in tissue repair, MSCs must be in close association with several stromal and immune cells. The mode of action of MSC tissue repair is complex wherein MSC-derived immunoregulatory factors play a critical role.

MSCs are reported to release an array of growth factors and immunomodulatory molecules (**Table 1**).

To investigate how the inflammatory microenvironment modulated secretion of anti-inflammatory factors at the sites of tissue damage and it was concluded that MSC-mediated immunosuppression occurs in the microenvironment surrounding the MSCs: the inflammatory factors produced during the immune response act to turn on the immunosuppressive capacity of MSCs. For example, during pregnancy, the developed immunological tolerance along with the fetus development highlights the key role of fetus-derived MSCs. These pleotropic cells inhibit a group of cells involved in innate and adaptive immunity such as B cells, dendritic cells (DC), macrophages, and various effector cells such as NK, CD4+ T, CD8+ T, regulatory T (Treg), and NKT cells [33, 34]. The contribution of MSC-derived molecules toward the immunoregulation has been discussed (**Figure 3**).

3.1 Indoleamine-2,3-dioxygenase (IDO)

Indoleamine-2,3-dioxygenase is a mammalian cytosolic enzyme responsible for catalyzing the initial step in tryptophan catabolism via the kynurenine degradation pathways. IDO is comprised of two alpha helical domains with a heme group located between them and is an essential amino acid which catalyzes the rate-limiting step in the degradation of tryptophan, with the kynurenine pathway [35]. Any reduction in the concentration of local tryptophan or its metabolite results in immunomodulatory effect by IDO expressing cells.

MSCs Secretome Profile	Functions
(a) MSCs Soluble factors	
HGF	T-cell inhibition
HLA-G5	T-cell inhibition/T reg expansion-NK
IDO	T-cell inhibition-NK inhibition
IGF	T-cell inhibition
IL1RA	T-cell inhibition-MF inhibition
IL-6	T-cell inhibition-DC inhibition
LIF	T-cell inhibition/T reg expansion
PGE-2	T-cell inhibition-NK inhibition
(b) MSCs membrane bound factors	
Jagged 1	T-cell inhibition
HLA-G1	T-cell inhibition/T reg expansion
PDL-1/PDL-2	T-cell inhibition
CD54	T reg expansion
CD58	T reg expansion
(c) Chemokines Factors	
CCR2, CCR3, CCR4, CCR5,CCR6,CCR7	Attractor; adhesion; transmigration
CXCR1, CXCR2, CXCR3, CXCR4, CXCR5	Recruitment, attraction, activation
Selectins	Tethering; rolling
VCAM	Arrest, adhesion, transmigration
SDF-1	regulates progenitor cell mobilization
(d) Growth Factors	
FGF	Induce angiogenesis (together with VEGF), has anti-apoptotic and anti-fibrotic effects,
VEGF	Induce angiogenesis, stimulate proliferation of peritubular capillaries, anti-apoptotic effects
TPO	Supports maintenance and proliferation of HSCs
SCF	Supports maintenance and proliferation of HSCs
HGF	Associated with mobilization of progenitor cells, induction of angiogenesis, improves cell growth, anti-apoptotic and anti-fibrotic effects
BDNF	Promotes survival and differentiation of neuronal tissue
MMP	Matrix and Growth Factor Degradation, Facilitate Cell Migration
PDGF	Tissue Repair
IGF-1	Wound Healing, Neurogenesis

Table 1.
Secretome profile of hMSCs and their functions.

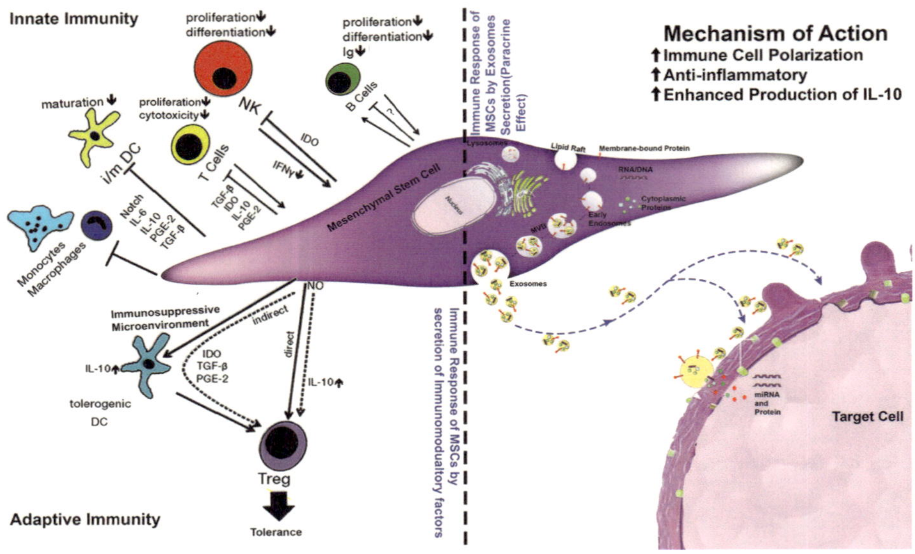

Figure 3.
Representative image shows the immune response of MSCs by secretion of IM factors (left panel). Immunoregulatory function of MSCs on different cell types of the innate and adaptive immune cells. (Right panel) paracrine effect of MSCs through secretion of exosomes and their fusion with the target cell membrane and release of the biological active content for immunomodulatory effect.

The studies carried out with placental cells showed that they are capable of preventing maternal T-cell destruction of the fetus during pregnancy, which happens due to the expression of IDO in placental cells. During pregnancy, the fetus expresses paternal antigens that do not provoke rejection by the mother like other semi-allogeneic grafts [36, 37]. Dendritic cells can also express IDO and thus induce a tolerogenic response. Su et al. suggest that MSCs do not have the innate ability to express IDO but gain this ability following stimulation by the pro-inflammatory cytokines IFN-γ and TNF-α in combination with IL-1β [38]. Recently, the role of IDO in MSC-mediated immunoregulation has been demonstrated in the suppression of various immune cell populations, including T cells and NK cells [39, 40].

3.2 Human leukocyte antigen-G (HLA-G)

HLA-G is a major histocompatibility complex class I antigen encoded by a gene on chromosome 6p21. It differs from classical HLA class I molecules by its restricted tissue distribution and limited polymorphism in the coding region. HLA-G can be expressed as seven distinct protein isoforms, each encoded by a specific, alternatively spliced transcript. Four isoforms are membrane-bound proteins (HLA-G1, HLA-G2, HLA-G3, and HLA-G4), and the other three isoforms are soluble proteins (HLA-G5, HLA-G6, and HLA-G7) [41]. It exerts its immunomodulatory functions by interacting with multiple receptors such as LILRB1(ILT2/CD85j), LILRB2 (ILT4/CD85d), and KIR2DL4 (CD158d) which are differentially expressed by immune cells. Besides these receptors, HLA-G can also bind to CD8 without T-cell receptor (TCR) interaction, provoking NK cells and activated CD8 + T cell-induced apoptosis as well as FASL upregulation and secretion [42, 43]. HLA-G plays a fundamental role in maternal tolerance and transplantation. HLA-G expression by MSCs can be positively modulated by IL-10 and leukemia inhibitory factor (LIF). Other molecules such as glucocorticoid and interferon-β (IFN-β) are found to regulate HLA-G expression in immune cells. HLA-G has been investigated for allogeneic solid organ transplantation and has been well associated with reduced number of immune rejection cases in kidney and liver allogeneic transplantations [44, 45].

3.3 Prostaglandin E2 (PGE-2)

Prostaglandins are small molecule derivatives of arachidonic acid (AA), produced by cyclooxygenase (COX, constitutively active cyclooxygenase COX1 and inducible COX2) and PG synthases. It can be produced by all cell types of the body, with epithelia, fibroblast, and infiltrating inflammatory cells representing the major sources of PGE-2 in the course of an immune response. The receptors of PGE2 (EP1–EP4) are present on multiple cell types, reflecting the ubiquitous function of PGE-2. It is relatively stable in vitro although its decay is accelerated by albumin [46]. In contrast, PGE-2 has a very rapid throughput rate in in vivo conditions and is quickly eliminated from tissues and circulation. This property of PGE-2 is most likely to contribute toward immune pathology and constitutes a potential target for immunomodulation. It is worth noting that the effect of PGE-2 in MSC-mediated immunoregulation in most cases is exerted in combination with other immunosuppressive molecules. With human MSCs, PGE-2 has been found to act with IDO to alter T-cell proliferation, during proliferation, cytotoxicity, and cytokine production by NK cells [47].

3.4 Inducible nitric oxide synthase (iNOs)

Nitric oxide synthases are family of enzymes catalyzing the production of nitric oxide from L-arginine. The enzymes convert arginine into citrulline and produce NO in the process. NO activity is independent of the level of calcium in the cell. However, its activity as other NO isoforms is dependent upon the binding of calmodulin (CaM). NO in high concentration is known to inhibit immune responses through mechanisms that remain largely unidentified. In addition, upon induction cytokines such as TNF-α and IFN-γ, alone or in combination, stimulate NO. This has a significant impact on both primary and secondary immune responses. For example, NO targets dendritic cells (DCs) that have a crucial role in making powerful immune response. It was found to prevent maturation of rat lung DCs by inhibiting granulocyte-macrophage colony-stimulating factors. Similarly, NO inhibits TNF-α and prevents DC maturation in humans [48]. MSCs produce large amounts of chemokines and adhesion molecules; immune cells accumulate in close proximity to the MSCs, where the high concentration of secreted NO can suppress the immune cells [49, 50].

3.5 Interleukin 10 (IL-10)

IL-10 is produced by both myeloid and lymphoid cells. While it is good immune suppressor, it has some immune stimulatory effects. IL-10 is recognized by its effect on T cells, macrophages, and monocytes which ultimately prohibit inflammatory responses. Thus, it regulates growth and differentiation of B cells, T cells, NK cells, and other cells of the immune system hence influencing inflammatory responses. IL-10 has the capability to inhibit the production of IL-2, TNF-α, IL-12, and IFN-γ. Furthermore, it will downregulate HLA class I. Although IL-10 has been implicated in MSC-mediated immunosuppression, direct IL-10 production by MSCs has not been demonstrated so far. Instead, contact of antigen-presenting cells such as dendritic cells or monocytes with MSCs has been found to induce IL-10 production [51–53].

3.6 Other mediators

In addition to the above molecules, several additional mediators are produced by MSCs or other adult stem/progenitor cells upon inflammatory stimulation, such as the inhibitory surface protein programmed death ligand 1 (PD-L1) [54], heme oxygenase-1 (HO-1) [55], leukemia inhibitory factor (LIF), galectins [56], and TGF-β [57]. However, their modes of action and underlying molecular mechanisms that drive MSC-mediated immunosuppression require further investigation.

3.7 Molecular and cellular interaction of MSCs with innate and acquired immune cells

3.7.1 MSC interaction with T and B cells

The antigen-specific immune system allows the development of immunological memory. It comprises of CD4+ T helper and CD8+ cytotoxic T lymphocytes that deliver a customized antigen-specific immune response following antigen processing and presentation by antigen-presenting cells (APCs). T helper cells comprise a subpopulation of cells called Tregs, which are specialized in suppression of T cell-mediated immune response [58]. The innate immune system plays an important role in the activation and subsequent course of adaptive immune response [59]. In addition, MSCs are able to suppress in vitro T-cell proliferation induced by cellular or non-specific mitogenic stimuli through the secretion of various soluble factors that include (transforming growth factor-beta 1) TGF-β, HGF, PGE-2, IDO, HLA-G5, and NO. The effect of these suppressive factors is upregulated by pre-sensitization of MSCs with TNF-α and IFN-γ. It is also known that MSCs polarize T cells toward a regulatory phenotype that serves as an important mechanism by which MSCs dampen inflammation [60, 61]. Tregs comprise a subpopulation of T helper cells, which are specialized in suppression of T cell-mediated immune response and characteristically express the forkhead box P3 (Fox P3) transcription factor. These are two main subsets of Tregs including a population of Fox P3+ natural Tregs which are thymus derived and specific for self-antigen and induced or adaptive Tregs that are derived from mature CD4 + CD35-FoxP3 precursors in the periphery following inflammatory stimuli. The in vitro co-culturing of MSCs with PBMNCs induced the differentiation of CD4+ T cells into CD25 + FoxP3+ expressing regulatory T cells [40, 62]. The possible reason of abovementioned mechanism is due to cell-cell contact of MSCs with helper T cells and secretion of PGE-2 and TGF-β. All together, these studies indicate that MSCs are able to maintain the balance between inflammatory effector T cells and anti-inflammatory Tregs.

B cells are also a major cell type involved in adaptive immune response, known for antigen presentation and antibody production. The balance between the different B-cell subsets has been identified as an important factor for optimal graft outcomes. To support the beneficial effect of B-cell depletion at the time of transplantation to impair T cell-mediated allo-response, the CD8 and CD4 T-cell memory is impaired when the antigen-presenting function of B cells is absent [63]. The exposure of enriched B-cell population to irradiated third party PBMNCs led to an increase in immunoglobulin (Ig) production that was abrogated by the addition of MSCs. There are diverse results among the studies to analyze the effect of MSCs upon exposure of isolated pure B cells [64]. These effects have been shown to be cell-cell contact independent or indirect through inhibition of pDC-induced B-cell maturation. On exposure, MSCs increased the viability of B cells and mediated the arrest of cell cycle at G0/G1 and inhibition of their differentiation into plasma cells and subsequent Ig formation, whereas it was observed that pre-treatment of

MSCs with IFN-γ was necessary for their suppressive effect on B cells [66]. The activated B cells and memory B-cell subsets when exposed to MSCs were seen to increase their survival and proliferation [65]. The studies carried out by Schu et al. [66] showed that when allogeneic MSCs were injected into rats, a strong humoral response was elicited as compared to injection with syngeneic cells in an immunocompetent host.

To support whether the allogeneic MSCs exert a humoral response in the recipient to prove the notion, they performed the experiment in which a rat was injected with allogeneic MSCs; on the other hand, contradictory reports were also published stating after transplantation none of them developed anti-MSC antibodies [66]. These studies indicate some disparity of humoral response directed against the injected MSCs, and possible reasons may be the source of MSCs, number of injected cells and frequency of injections, route of administration, or concurrent immunosuppression used.

3.7.2 MSC interaction with NK cells

Natural killer cells or NK cells are a type of cytotoxic lymphocytes critical to the innate immune system, evolve as progenitors in the bone marrow, and circulate as mature cells in the blood. They provide rapid responses to viral-infected cells, acting 3 days after infection, and respond to tumor formation. They play a major role in the mechanisms of rejection of graft and are central to the regulation of cytotoxicity in response to human leukocyte antigen molecule. With increasing trends in therapeutic usage of MSCs for treatment of GvHD, it is important to investigate the underlying effects of interaction of MSC and NK cells. They function in the manner that they get activated and inhibited on cell surface because of receptors transmitting the signal into the cell. Usually, NK cell possesses regulatory functions and can secrete cytokines and chemokines which modulate the host's immune response. IL-12 is the most important pro-inflammatory factor which responds to penetrating pathogens and acts through its high affinity receptors. It is released from accessory cells like monocytes, macrophages, and dendritic cells (DCs). Also, the most important cytokine released by NK cells is IFN-γ which is produced upon stimulation of IL-12. The NK cell-derived IFN-y reinforces the expression of IL-12 and DCs via feedback mechanism. BM-MSCs directly interfere with the proliferation, cytokine production, and in some cases cytotoxicity of NK cells. MSC-NK interactions are complex and largely dependent on the microenvironment and activation status of the NK cells. Mainly, MSCs suppress the production of IL-2, IL-15, and INF-γ but not the cytotoxicity of freshly isolated NK cells. In addition, when activated NK cells come into contact with the MSCs, it interferes with NK-mediated cytotoxicity which is primarily mediated by cell-cell contact and secretion of IDO, PGE-2, TGF-β1, and HLA-G5. Other reports mentioned that when licensed MSCs were exposed to IFN-γ, they are protected from NK-mediated cell killing, potentially due to their upregulated cell surface expression of HLA-I and downregulation of ULBP-3. This alongside an increased production of both IDO and PGE-2 offers multiple mechanisms for dampening NK responsiveness to the MSCs [59, 67, 68].

3.7.3 MSC interaction with dendritic cells

The potent antigen-presenting cells (APCs) and dendritic cells (DCs) play a pivotal role in initiating immune response. The life span of DCs can be divided into two major phases, an immature stage and a mature stage. These phases can be differentiated further on the basis of molecules expressed (CD80, CD86, OX62, HLA-II, and CD11b/c) on their surface. DCs can be immunostimulatory or immunosuppressive, depending upon their maturation stage and specific DC subset. Immature DCs (iDCs) express low levels of HLA-II but no co-stimulatory molecules. The interaction of MSCs with DCs leads to the inhibition of maturation of monocytes and CD34+ precursor cells. Moreover, the direct activation of DCs leads to the release of PGE-2, IL-6, TSG-6, MCSF, and jagged-2 mediated signaling. Tolerogenic phenotype occurs when DC secretome of pro-inflammatory cytokines (TNF-α and IL-12) shifts toward anti-inflammatory IL-10 in which further downstream induces Th2 and Treg responses [69–71].

4. Paracrine interaction with in the niche (exosomes)

Advances in stem cell technology have opened interesting perspectives within the realm of regenerative medicine. As reported, MSCs participate in repair and regenerative processes via different mechanisms like homing and transdifferentiation and immunomodulation, which depends on paracrine mechanisms [72, 73]. The initial studies using MSCs were based on local engrafting of MSCs and differentiating into multiple tissue types. However, with the in-depth study of different mechanisms of MSC action, it has been reported that <1% MSCs are able to survive transiently after systemic administration [74]. This suggests that paracrine mechanisms through secretion of various molecules called secretome might be the possible mechanism for MSC regenerative potential. This has attracted significant attention for the potential use of MSC secretome in tissue repair and regeneration.

The secretome released by MSCs includes various biologically active growth factors and cytokines which aid in immunomodulatory properties of MSCs [75]. However, we cannot neglect the fact that the secretome released in the milieu of ECM of the cells is an easy target for denaturation due to the presence of proteases and other enzymes in the microenvironmental niche. Therefore, these growth factors and cytokines have been shown to be packed into small vesicles called exosomes which are secreted by MSCs in the extracellular milieu of cell along with the secretome [76]. They function through encapsulation of biological active molecules such as miRNA, proteins, and immunomodulatory molecules and protect them from degradation.

4.1 Exosome formation to secretion

Exosomes are lipid membrane-bound extracellular vesicles which possess a diameter of 30–120 nm and a density of 1.09–1.18 g/mL and are secreted by all cell types. These exosomes carry cellular components like proteins and nucleic acids and aid in cell-cell communication. The exosome was first discovered in 1984 by Johnstone in sheep reticulocytes [77]. It was initially believed that exosomes remove unwanted proteins from cells. Later on, it was demonstrated that many other cell types also secrete exosomes including immune cells, cancer cells, stem cells, and many more [78].

Exosomes are endosomal in origin, formed within multivesicular endosomes (MVEs). These vesicles are being released when membranes of MVEs fuse with that of the cellular plasma membrane. These exosomes express various surface markers like CD63, CD81, and CD9. They carry surface molecules that are present on the parent cell which aids in identification of exosomes and their parent cell source as well [77].

Moreover, the exosomes secreted by stem cells carry various proteins (growth factors and cytokines) and nucleic acids (mRNA and miRNA) that can influence their mode of action [79]. The content carried by these vesicles depends on the type of cell (including source of cells) and its state of activation. Once released, these vesicles have local as well as remote effect by interacting with the neighboring cells or by circulating in the body fluids (bloodstream, saliva, serum, etc.).

4.2 Exosomes and immune cells

The exosomes were studied for their multifaceted application in antigen presentation, and vastly studied immune cell was dendritic cells. The clinical studies have been conducted to evaluate the dendritic cell derived exosomes for their therapeutic potential. However, compared to preclinical studies, only a few clinical trials have been conducted using exosomes. Reported studies were conducted where dendritic cell-derived exosomes were evaluated for their safety, tolerability, and efficacy in cancer patients. Exosomes carry parental cell surface marker expression. In this regard, DC derived exosomes are HLA-II positive as a result they can only be used in patient specific studies [80, 81]. In contrast, MSCs are immunologically naïve as they express only HLA class I molecules and lack HLA class II, CD40, CD80 and CD86 expression on their cell surface. Also, they are capable of immune escape and fail to induce an immune response by the transplanted host. Similarly, exosomes secreted by them are also immunologically naïve [82]. Considering all of the above properties, several recent studies have focused their research on evaluation of stem cell-derived exosomes in the area of immunomodulation with fewer reports.

In a recent study, exosomes derived from MSCs were specifically identified to mimic the effect of MSCs, and this paved the way to cell-free therapeutic approach using exosomes instead of the cell itself [83]. The first report using MSC exosomes were in cardiovascular diseases where Lai et al. [85] identified exosomes as the cardioprotective components in MSC paracrine secretion [84]. This was followed by several other studies where exosomes isolated from tissue-specific MSCs were studied for their therapeutic potential in various diseases.

Initial studies were performed on bone marrow-derived exosomes for evaluating their regenerative potential in cardiovascular diseases [85], acute kidney injury [86], bone defects, etc. [87]. By 2013, only researchers started exploring the regenerative potential of exosomes derived from adipose tissue and Wharton's jelly sources. These studies have explored the various mechanisms by which these exosomes mimic MSCs. The content of these exosomes was evaluated by using various techniques like RNA sequencing, mass spectrometry, etc., to identify different molecules and their target effect.

Conforti et al. reported the effect of MSC-derived vesicles on B-cell proliferation which was further confirmed by Di Trapani's group in 2016 [88, 89] . They observed that exosomes had higher levels of miRNAs compared to MSCs and induce inflammatory priming via increasing levels of miR-155 and miR-146. These are two miRNAs involved in the activation and inhibition of inflammatory reactions. Similar studies were reported where MSC-derived exosomes were shown to increase the ratio between regulatory and effector T cells along with the increase in cytokine such as IL-10 [90]. Similarly, Chen et al. [91] has also reported immunomodulatory effects of MSC-derived exosomes toward peripheral blood mononuclear cells (PBMNCs) focusing specifically on T cells. It was observed that there was significant inhibition of pro-inflammatory cytokines, IL-1β and TNF-α, but enhancement of the expression of anti-inflammatory cytokine, TGF-β1. This cytokine profile in their study mimics the immunomodulatory effect of MSCs [91]. Zhang et al. showed that these exosomes may polarize monocytes toward M2-like phenotype, which in turn induces CD4+ T-cell differentiation into regulatory T cells [92].

Blazquez et al. demonstrated AD-MSC-derived exosomes as a therapeutic agent for the treatment of inflammation-related diseases. They showed that exosomes exerted an inhibitory effect on the differentiation of activated T cells, reduced T-cell proliferation, and IFN-γ secretion in an in vitro stimulated T-cell model [93]. Favaro et al. has shown the effect of BM-MSC-derived exosomes on PBMNCs isolated from type I diabetic patients. These exosomes were able to inhibit the IFN-γ production and significantly increased the production of immunomodulatory mediators such as PGE-2, TGF-β, IL-10, and IL-6 [94]. The in vitro studies were complemented by the in vivo studies which confirmed the immunosuppressive effect of exosomes in mouse allogeneic skin grafting models [95]. Bai et al 2017 have subcutaneously administered exosomes isolated from human embryonic stem cell-derived MSCs and showed that there was delayed occurrence of GvHD for 2 days, concomitant with increasing Treg polarization. In continuation, the author has also demonstrated that exosomes released from WJ-MSCs can effectively ameliorate experimental autoimmune uveoretinitis (EAU) in rats by inhibiting the migration of inflammatory cells [95]. Moreover, there is only single case study on humans in which MSC exosomes have been tested in the treatment of resistant grade IV acute GvHD patient which experienced improvement in symptoms for 5 months. There were no side effects reported, and the decrease of pro-inflammatory cytokines such as TNF-α, IL-1β, and IFN-γ was observed. The anti-inflammatory molecules IL-10, TGF-β1, and HLA-G contained in the exosome preparations were believed to contribute to the immunosuppressive effect of MSC-Exo [96].

Although there are limited studies available using MSC-derived exosomes, future advancements into research and gain in in-depth knowledge of immunomodulatory properties of these MSC exosomes could be seen. These nano-vesicles can be developed as cell-free therapies. The use of these exosomes as cell-free therapies provides following key advantages:

a. Less tumorigenicity.

b. Easy storage without application of potentially toxic cryopreservative agents.

c. Mass production through tailor-made cell lines.

d. Potential to be used as ready-to-go biologic product.

e. Off-the-shelf secretome therapies.

f. The time and cost of expansion and maintenance could be greatly reduced.

g. The biological product obtained could be modified to desired cell-specific effects.

Despite these advantages of MSC-derived exosomes, there has been a lack of manufacturing process that is required to generate exosomes with clinically relevant quantities. Therefore, there is an urgent need for technological advancements. Nevertheless, regulatory requirements will be necessary to establish the safety and efficacy profile of these exosome products.

5. MSCs in preclinical and clinical trials

MSCs delivered alone or with a biomaterial have been used in a variety of regenerative medicine strategies. In vivo evidence supports the hypothesis that MSCs have immunosuppressive properties that include prevention of graft versus host disease (GvHD), decreased graft rejection, prevention of experimental acute encephalomyelitis, prolonged skin graft survival, etc. [8]. However, in recent years, consistent reports on its immunomodulatory properties have opened up newer avenues for studying MSCs, other than regenerative medicine. As of May 2018, there were over 843 MSC-related clinical trials registered on the NIH Clinical Trial Database (http://clinicaltrial.gov/). Interestingly, half of all registered clinical trials (~45%) are being conducted for immune-mediated diseases. Of these, 69 are based on autoimmune disease, 38 on GVHD, and the rest 290 on other inflammatory diseases. However, in early phase I, phase II, phase III, and phase IV, there were 3, 76, 7, and 6 clinical trials conducted, respectively. Hematopoietic stem cells (HSCs) have been the most successful in providing therapeutic application using stem cells. MSCs represent a lifesaving treatment for patients suffering with hematopoietic malignancies and genetic diseases. HSC transplantation is performed either autologous or with matched allogeneic/third party, depending upon the clinical scenario. Furthermore, in allogenic transplantation, immunosuppression is necessary to reduce the graft rejection in patients. But despite immunosuppressant therapy, immune rejection in the form of GvHD is still a major cause of morbidity and mortality. The clinical application of MSCs for GvHD developed more rapidly than for any other immune-mediated diseases [68]. The probable cause could be case reports in severe GvHD where BMSCs were infused and showed dramatic therapeutic effects. Clearly, MSCs have a strong potential as therapeutic agents for GvHD, but detailed tailoring of patient population and stringent MSC processing criteria are necessary to deliver consistent and reproducible results [97–100].

Apart from GvHD condition, multiple sclerosis (MS), joint diseases such as osteoarthritis (OA) and rheumatoid arthritis (RA), inflammatory bowel diseases (IBD) and inflammatory airway, and pulmonary diseases are few examples of inflammatory diseases in which preclinical studies have established strong therapeutic effect of MSCs [101]. In multiple sclerosis, reports showed that MSC treatment increases accumulation of Th2 cytokines-IL-4 and IL-5 and generation of Treg in vivo both of which help reduce EAE symptomatology. The possible molecular mechanism by which MSCs polarize CD4 T cells in EAE is via IDO. Indeed, both small and large animal studies demonstrate that MSCs decrease inflammation in joint diseases and facilitate cartilage repair [102].

The critical part of IBD is the uncontrolled immune response to intestinal microbes, and it is progressively fatal without curative treatment, making MSCs an attractive therapeutic option for these chronic inflammatory diseases. In several experimental models of IBD, MSCs given by intraperitoneal or intravenous routes showed prevention of DSS-induced injury of the intestines. It was observed that MSCs can specifically reduce Th1 and Th17 responses as well as serum level of pro-inflammatory cytokines (IL-1b, IL-6, IL-17, TNF-α, and IFN-γ) while enhancing the numbers of Tregs and splenic (myeloid-derived suppressor cells) MDSCs. A very recent trial using allogeneic placenta-derived MSC-like cells (which were not registered) also showed favorable immune responses. Thus, MSC therapy for IBD—especially CD fistula formation—appears to be safe and a viable option [103, 104].

Pulmonary diseases like chronic obstructive lung disease (COPD) are driven by alveolar macrophages, cytotoxic T cells, and neutrophils leading to progressive limitations in airflow with small airway fibrosis and alveolar destruction. In in vivo studies documented post-MSC infusion showed downregulation of pro-inflammatory cytokines such as TNF-α, IL-1β, and IL-6 and upregulation of VEGF and TGF-β [105, 106]. In addition, MSCs or MSC-conditioned medium improved tissue damage and survival. This involves MSC-derived factors with microvesicles such as exosomes, which are considered as carriers.

6. Conclusion

MSCs are excellent candidates for therapeutic use as cellular therapies can potentially revolutionize the current pharmaceutical landscape. Emerging data suggests that MSCs have an immunomodulatory function, but thorough understanding of the mechanisms underlying the complex molecular interplay between MSCs and inflammatory responses will be crucial for exploiting MSC-based therapies in therapeutic applications. One important aspect is to delineate functional differences in tissue-specific MSCs isolated from different sources; current ISCT standardization does not include immune-related functional tests or more detailed molecular validation. Based on the evidence of several clinical trials, the safety of this therapy appears clear; however, the efficacy of such cell therapy is largely uncertain. The overwhelming positive results seen in preclinical animal studies have not yet been translated into clinic. In brief, there is still much to learn, explore, and optimize with regard to the interactions of MSCs in human pathological conditions. In the near future, based on current development and results, MSCs are expected to hold tremendous potential to achieve clinical relevance in regenerative therapy.

Acknowledgements

The authors would like to thank Mr. Manish Prajapati, for his expert help in designing the graphics for this book chapter. Authors would also like to thank Dr. Rituparna Chaudhari and Dr. Swati Midha for their critical evaluation of this book chapter.

Conflict of interest

The authors declare that they have no competing interest.

Abbreviations

ESC	embryonic stem cell
ASC	adult stem cell
MSC	mesenchymal stem cell
ISCT	International Society for Cellular Therapy
HLA	human leukocyte antigen
NK Cells	natural killer cells
BM-MSCs	bone marrow-derived MSCs
AD-MSCs	adipose tissue-derived MSCs
WJ-MSCs	Wharton's jelly-derived MSCs
INF-γ	interferon gamma
TNF-α	tumor necrosis factor-α
IL-1	interleukin-1
HCELL	hematopoietic cell E-/L-selectin ligand
ECM	extracellular matrix
VCAM1	vascular cell adhesion molecule-1
VL4	very late antigen-4
MMP	matrix metalloproteinases
TIMP-3	tissue inhibitor of metalloproteinases 3
NKT	natural killer T cell

DC	dendritic cells
Treg	regulatory T cells
IDO	indoleamine-2,3-dioxygenase
HLA-G	human leukocyte antigen-G
LILRB1	leukocyte immunoglobulin-like receptor B1
LILRB2	leukocyte immunoglobulin-like receptor B2
KIR2DL4	killer cell immunoglobulin like receptor
TCR	T-cell receptor
IFN-beta	interferon-B
PGE-2	prostaglandin E2
AA	arachidonic acid
COX	cyclooxygenase
iNOs	inducible nitric oxide synthase
CaM	calmodulin
PD-L1	protein programmed death ligand 1
HO-1	heme oxygenase-1
LIF	leukemia inhibitory factor
APCs	antigen-presenting cells
TGF-β1	transforming growth factor-beta 1
HGF	hepatocyte growth factor
FoxP3	forkhead box P3
PBMNCs	peripheral blood mononuclear cells
Ig	immunoglobulin
GvHD	graft versus host disease
ULBP-3	UL16-binding protein 3 (ULBP3)
MVEs	multivesicular endosomes
EAU	autoimmune uveoretinitis
HSCs	hematopoietic stem cells
MS	multiple sclerosis
OA	osteoarthritis
RA	rheumatoid arthritis
IBD	inflammatory bowel diseases
EAE	experimental autoimmune encephalomyelitis
COPD	chronic obstructive lung disease
VEGF	vascular endothelial growth factor

Author details

Sonali Rawat, Suchi Gupta and Sujata Mohanty*
Stem Cell Facility, DBT-Centre of Excellence for Stem Cell Research, AIIMS, New Delhi, India

*Address all correspondence to: drmohantysujata@gmail.com

References

[1] Davies JE, Walker JT, Keating A. Concise review: Wharton's jelly: The rich, but enigmatic, source of mesenchymal stromal cells. Stem Cells Translational Medicine. 2017;**6**(7):1620-1630

[2] El Omar R, Beroud J, Stoltz J-F, Menu P, Velot E, Decot V. Umbilical cord mesenchymal stem cells: The new gold standard for mesenchymal stem cell-based therapies? Tissue Engineering. Part B, Reviews. 2014;**20**(5):523-544

[3] Kwon A et al. Tissue-specific differentiation potency of mesenchymal stromal cells from perinatal tissues. Scientific Reports. 2016;**6**:1-11

[4] Chen JY, Mou XZ, Du XC, Xiang C. Comparative analysis of biological characteristics of adult mesenchymal stem cells with different tissue origins. Asian Pacific Journal of Tropical Medicine. 2015;**8**(9):739-746

[5] Paliwal S, Chaudhuri R, Agrawal A, Mohanty S. Regenerative abilities of mesenchymal stem cells through mitochondrial transfer. Journal of Biomedical Science. 2018;**25**(1):31

[6] Billing AM et al. Comprehensive transcriptomic and proteomic characterization of human mesenchymal stem cells reveals source specific cellular markers. Scientific Reports. 2016;**6**(2):1-15

[7] Dominici M et al. Minimal criteria for defining multipotent mesenchymal stromal cells. The International Society for Cellular Therapy position statement. Cytotherapy. 2006;**8**(4):315-317

[8] Alagesan S, Griffin MD. Autologous and allogeneic mesenchymal stem cells in organ transplantation: What do we know about their safety and efficacy? Current Opinion in Organ Transplantation. 2014;**19**(1):65-72

[9] Honczarenko M, Le Y, Swierkowski M, Ghiran I, Glodek AM, Silberstein LE. Human bone marrow stromal cells express a distinct set of biologically functional chemokine receptors. Stem Cells. 2006;**24**(4):1030-1041

[10] Kinkaid HYM, Huang X-P, Li R-K, Weisel RD. What's new in cardiac cell therapy? Allogeneic bone marrow stromal cells as 'universal donor' cells. Journal of Cardiac Surgery. 2010;**25**(3):359-366

[11] Atoui R, Chiu RCJ. Concise review: Immunomodulatory properties of mesenchymal stem cells in cellular transplantation: Update, controversies, and unknowns. Stem Cells Translational Medicine. 2012;**1**(3):200-205

[12] Agematsu K, Nakahori Y. Recipient origin of bone marrow-derived fibroblastic stromal cells during all periods following bone marrow transplantation in humans. British Journal of Haematology. 1991;**79**(3):359-365

[13] Medzhitov R. Inflammation 2010: New adventures of an old flame. Cell. 2010;**140**(6):771-776

[14] Krysko DV et al. Macrophages use different internalization mechanisms to clear apoptotic and necrotic cells. Cell Death and Differentiation. 2006;**13**(12):2011-2022

[15] Han Z, Jing Y, Zhang S, Liu Y, Shi Y, Wei L. The role of immunosuppression of mesenchymal stem cells in tissue repair and tumor growth. Cell & Bioscience. 2012;**2**(1):8

[16] Kalinina NI, Sysoeva VY, Rubina KA, Parfenova YV, Tkachuk VA. Mesenchymal stem cells in tissue growth and repair. Acta Naturae. 2011;**3**(4):30-37

[17] Segers VFM et al. Regulation and function of stem cells in the cardiovascular system mesenchymal stem cell adhesion to cardiac microvascular endothelium: Activators and mechanisms. System. 2006:1370-1377

[18] Rüster B et al. Mesenchymal stem cells display coordinated rolling and adhesion behavior on endothelial cells mesenchymal stem cells display coordinated rolling and adhesion behavior on endothelial cells. Blood. 2008;**108**(12):3938-3944

[19] Sackstein R. The bone marrow is akin to skin: HCELL and the biology of hematopoietic stem cell homing. The Journal of Investigative Dermatology. 2004;**122**(5):1061-1069

[20] Sackstein R et al. Ex vivo glycan engineering of CD44 programs human multipotent mesenchymal stromal cell trafficking to bone. Nature Medicine. 2008;**14**(2):181-187

[21] Ip JE, Wu Y, Huang J, Zhang L, Pratt RE, Dzau VJ. Mesenchymal stem cells use integrin 1 not CXC chemokine receptor 4 for myocardial migration and engraftment. Molecular Biology of the Cell. 2007;**18**:2873-2882

[22] Popov C et al. Integrins α2β1 and α11β1 regulate the survival of mesenchymal stem cells on collagen i. Cell Death & Disease. 2011;**2**(7):e186-e113

[23] Steingen C, Brenig F, Baumgartner L, Schmidt J, Schmidt A, Bloch W. Characterization of key mechanisms in transmigration and invasion of mesenchymal stem cells. Journal of Molecular and Cellular Cardiology. 2008;**44**(6):1072-1084

[24] Koç ON et al. Bone marrow-derived mesenchymal stem cells remain host-derived despite successful hematopoietic engraftment after allogeneic transplantation in patients with lysosomal and peroxisomal storage diseases. Experimental Hematology. 1999;**27**(11):1675-1681

[25] Santucci MA et al. Host origin of bone marrow fibroblasts following allogeneic bone marrow transplantation for chronic myeloid leukemia. Bone Marrow Transplantation. 1992;**10**(3):255-259

[26] Caplan AI. The mesengenic process. Clinics in Plastic Surgery. 1994;**21**:429-435

[27] Almeida-Porada G, Porada CD, Tran N, Zanjani ED. Cotransplantation of human stromal cell progenitors into preimmune fetal sheep results in early appearance of human donor cells in circulation and boosts cell levels in bone marrow at later time points after transplantation. Blood. 2000;**95**(11):3620-3627

[28] Liechty KW et al. Human mesenchymal stem cells engraft and demonstrate site-specific differentiation after in utero transplantation in sheep. Nature Medicine. 2000;**6**:1282

[29] Gao J, Dennis JE, Muzic RF, Lundberg M, Caplan AI. The dynamic in vivo distribution of bone marrow-derived mesenchymal stem cells after infusion. Cells, Tissues, Organs. 2001;**169**(1):12-20

[30] Bentzon JF et al. Tissue distribution and engraftment of human mesenchymal stem cells immortalized by human telomerase reverse transcriptase gene. Biochemical and Biophysical Research Communications. 2005;**330**(3):633-640

[31] Karen E. Mechanisms of mesenchymal stromal cell immunomodulation. Immunology and Cell Biology. 2012;**91**(1):19-26

[32] Fridman R. Matrix metalloproteinases. Biochimica et

Biophysica Acta, Molecular Cell Research. 2010;**1803**(1):1-2

[33] Wang M, Yuan Q, Xie L. Mesenchymal Stem Cell-Based Immunomodulation: Properties and Clinical Application. Stem cells international. 2018:3057624. DOI: 10.1155/2018/3057624

[34] Duffy MM, Ritter T, Ceredig R, Griffin MD. Mesenchymal stem cell effects on T-cell effector pathways. Stem Cell Research & Therapy. 2011;**2**(4):1-9

[35] Takikawa O, Kuroiwa T, Yamazaki F, Kido R. Mechanism of interferon-γ action. Characterization of indoleamine 2,3-dioxygenase in cultured human cells induced by interferon -γ and evaluation of the enzyme-mediated tryptophan degradation in its anticellular activity. The Journal of Biological Chemistry. 1988;**263**(4):2041-2048

[36] Mellor AL et al. Indoleamine 2, 3-dioxygenase, immunosuppression and pregnancy. Journal of Reproductive Immunology. 2002;**57**(1-2):143-150

[37] Munn DH et al. GCN2 kinase in T cells mediates proliferative arrest and anergy induction in response to indoleamine 2,3-dioxygenase. Immunity. 2005;**22**(5):633-642

[38] Su J et al. Phylogenetic distinction of iNOS and IDO function in mesenchymal stem cell-mediated immunosuppression in mammalian species. Cell Death and Differentiation. 2014;**21**(3):388-396

[39] Meisel R, Zibert A, Laryea M, Göbel U, Däubener W, Dilloo D. Human bone marrow stromal cells inhibit allogeneic T-cell responses by indoleamine 2,3-dioxygenase–mediated tryptophan degradation. Blood. 2004;**103**(12):4619-4621

[40] English K, Ryan JM, Tobin L, Murphy MJ, Barry FP, Mahon BP. Cell contact, prostaglandin E_2 and transforming growth factor beta 1 play non-redundant roles in human mesenchymal stem cell induction of $CD4^+$ $CD25^{High}$ forkhead box $P3^+$ regulatory T cells. Clinical and Experimental Immunology. 2009;**156**(1):149-160

[41] Carosella ED, Paul P, Moreau P, Rouas-Freiss N. HLA-G and HLA-E: Fundamental and pathophysiological aspects. Immunology Today. 2000;**21**(11):532-534

[42] Rajagopalan S, Long EO. A human histocompatibility leukocyte antigen (HLA)-G-specific receptor expressed on all natural killer cells. The Journal of Experimental Medicine. 1999;**189**(7):1093-1100

[43] Selmani Z et al. Human leukocyte antigen-G5 secretion by human mesenchymal stem cells is required to suppress T lymphocyte and natural killer function and to induce $CD4^+$ $CD25^{high}$ $FOXP3^+$ regulatory T cells. Stem Cells. 2008;**26**(1):212-222

[44] Lefebvre S et al. Molecular mechanisms controlling constitutive and IFN-gamma-inducible HLA-G expression in various cell types. Journal of Reproductive Immunology. 1999;**43**(2):213-224

[45] Moreau P et al. IL-10 selectively induces HLA-G expression in human trophoblasts and monocytes. International Immunology. 1999;**11**(5):803-811

[46] Hata AN, Breyer RM. Pharmacology and signaling of prostaglandin receptors: Multiple roles in inflammation and immune modulation. Pharmacology & Therapeutics. 2004;**103**(2):147-166

[47] Spaggiari GM, Capobianco A, Abdelrazik H, Becchetti F, Mingari MC, Moretta L. Mesenchymal stem cells

inhibit natural killer cell proliferation, cytotoxicity , and cytokine production: Role of indoleamine 2, 3-dioxygenase and prostaglandin E2. Blood. 2008;**111**(3):1327-1333

[48] Serbina NV, Salazar-Mather TP, Biron CA, Kuziel WA, Pamer EG. TNF/iNOS-producing dendritic cells mediate innate immune defense against bacterial infection. Immunity. 2003;**19**(1):59-70

[49] Bogdan C. Nitric oxide and the immune response. Nature Immunology. 2001;**2**(10):907-916

[50] Porterfield DM et al. Proteins and lipids define the diffusional field of nitric oxide. American Journal of Physiology. Lung Cellular and Molecular Physiology. 2001;**281**(4):L904-L912

[51] Matsuda M et al. Interleukin 10 pretreatment protects target cells from tumor- and allo-specific cytotoxic T cells and downregulates HLA class I expression. The Journal of Experimental Medicine. 1994;**180**(6):2371-2376

[52] Moore KW, de Waal Malefyt R, Coffman RL, O'Garra A. Interleukin −10 and the INterleukin −10 REceptor. Annual Review of Immunology. 2001;**19**(1):683-765

[53] Németh K, Leelahavanichkul A, Yuen PS, et al. Bone marrow stromal cells attenuate sepsis via prostaglandin E(2)-dependent reprogramming of host macrophages to increase their interleukin-10 production. Nat Med. 2008;**15**(1):42-49

[54] Sheng H et al. A critical role of IFNγ in priming MSC-mediated suppression of T cell proliferation through up-regulation of B7-H1. Cell Research. 2008;**18**(8):846-857

[55] Maines MD. Heme oxygenase: Function, multiplicity, regulatory mechanisms, and clinical applications. The FASEB Journal. 1988;**2**(10):557-2568

[56] Sioud M, Mobergslien A, Boudabous A, Fløisand Y. Mesenchymal stem cell-mediated T cell suppression occurs through secreted galectins. International Journal of Oncology. 2011;**38**(2):385-390

[57] Moore AG et al. The transforming growth factor-β superfamily cytokine macrophage inhibitory cytokine-1 is present in high concentrations in the serum of pregnant women. The Journal of Clinical Endocrinology and Metabolism. 2000;**85**(12):4781-4788

[58] Eller K, Rosenkranz AR. Specialized Regulatory T Cells for Optimal Suppression of T Cell Responses in GN. Journal American Society of Nephrology. 2016;**28**(1):1-2

[59] Noone C, Kihm A, English K, O'Dea S, Mahon BP. IFN-γ stimulated human umbilical-tissue-derived cells potently suppress NK activation and resist NK-mediated cytotoxicity in vitro. Stem Cells and Development. 2013;**22**(22):3003-3014

[60] Burr SP, Dazzi F, Garden OA. Mesenchymal stromal cells and regulatory T cells: The Yin and Yang of peripheral tolerance. Immunology and Cell Biology. 2013;**91**(1):12-18

[61] Chaudhry A, Rudensky AY. Control of inflammation by integration of environmental cues by regulatory T cells. The Journal of Clinical Investigation. 2013;**123**(3):939-944

[62] Maccario R et al. Interaction of human mesenchymal stem cells with cells involved in alloantigen-specific immune response favors the differentiation of CD4 + T-cell subsets expressing a regulatory/suppressive phenotype. Haematologica. 2005;**90**(4):516-525

[63] Ng Y-H, Oberbarnscheidt MH, Chandramoorthy HCK, Hoffman R, Chalasani G. B cells help alloreactive T cells differentiate into memory T cells. American Journal of Transplantation. 2010;**10**(9):1970-1980

[64] Comoli P et al. Human mesenchymal stem cells inhibit antibody production induced in vitro by allostimulation. Nephrology, Dialysis, Transplantation. 2008;**23**(4):1196-1202

[65] Schena F et al. Interferon-γ-dependent inhibition of B cell activation by bone marrow-derived mesenchymal stem cells in a murine model of systemic lupus erythematosus. Arthritis and Rheumatism. 2010;**62**(9):2776-2786

[66] Schu S et al. Immunogenicity of allogeneic mesenchymal stem cells. Journal of Cellular and Molecular Medicine. 2012;**16**(9):2094-2103

[67] Moretta A et al. Receptors for Hla class-I molecules in human natural killer cells. Annual Review of Immunology. 1996;**14**(1):619-648

[68] Spaggiari GM, Capobianco A, Becchetti S, Mingari MC, Moretta L. Mesenchymal stem cell – Natural killer cell interactions: Evidence that activated NK cells are capable of killing MSCs, whereas MSCs can inhibit IL-2 – Induced NK-cell proliferation. Blood. 2006;**107**(4):1484-1490

[69] Su WR, Zhang QZ, Shi SH, Nguyen AL, Le AD. Human gingiva-derived mesenchymal stromal cells attenuate contact hypersensitivity via prostaglandin E2-dependent mechanisms. Stem Cells. 2011;**29**(11):1849-1860

[70] Nauta AJ, Kruisselbrink AB, Lurvink E, Willemze R, Fibbe WE. Mesenchymal stem cells inhibit generation and function of both CD34+–derived and monocyte-derived dendritic cells. Journal of Immunology. 2006;**177**(4):2080-2087

[71] Liu Y et al. MSCs inhibit bone marrow-derived DC maturation and function through the release of TSG-6. Biochemical and Biophysical Research Communications. 2014;**450**(4):1409-1415

[72] Wang J et al. Role of mesenchymal stem cells, their derived factors, and extracellular vesicles in liver failure. Stem Cell Research & Therapy. 2017;**8**(1):137

[73] Fierabracci A, Del Fattore A, Luciano R, Muraca M, Teti A, Muraca M. Recent advances in mesenchymal stem cell immunomodulation: The role of microvesicles. Cell Transplantation. 2015;**24**(2):133-149

[74] Li L, Chen X, Wang WE, Zeng C. How to improve the survival of transplanted mesenchymal st cell in ischemic heart? Stem Cells International. 2016;**2016**(2):9682757

[75] Kesimer M et al. Characterization of exosome-like vesicles released from human tracheobronchial ciliated epithelium: A possible role in innate defense. The FASEB Journal. 2009;**23**(6):1858-1868

[76] Lai R, Chen T, Lim S. Mesenchymal stem cell exosome: A novel stem cell-based therapy for cardiovascular disease. Regenerative Medicine. 2011:481-492

[77] Yu B, Zhang X, Li X. Exosomes derived from mesenchymal stem cells. International Journal of Molecular Sciences. 2014;**15**(3):4142-4157

[78] Gong M et al. Mesenchymal stem cells release exosomes that transfer miRNAs to endothelial cells and promote angiogenesis. Oncotarget. 2017;**8**(28):45200-45212

[79] Cheng X et al. Mesenchymal stem cells deliver exogenous miR-21 via exosomes to inhibit nucleus pulposus cell apoptosis and reduce intervertebral disc degeneration. Journal of Cellular and Molecular Medicine. 2018;**22**(1):261-276

[80] Vincent-Schneider H et al. Exosomes bearing HLA-DR1 molecules need dendritic cells to efficiently stimulate specific T cells. International Immunology. 2002;**14**:713-722

[81] Barros FM, Carneiro F, Machado JC, Melo SA. Exosomes and immune response in cancer: Friends or foes? Frontiers in Immunology. 2018;**9**:730

[82] Ong S-G, Wu JC. Exosomes as potential alternatives to stem cell therapy in mediating cardiac regeneration. Circulation Research. 2015;**117**(1):7 LP-9 LP

[83] Phinney DG, Pittenger MF. Concise review: MSC-derived exosomes for cell-free therapy. Stem Cells. 2017;**35**(4):851-858

[84] Vizoso FJ, Eiro N, Cid S, Schneider J, Perez-Fernandez R. Mesenchymal stem cell secretome: Toward cell-free therapeutic strategies in regenerative medicine. International Journal of Molecular Sciences. 2017;**18**(9):1852

[85] Lai RC et al. Exosome secreted by MSC reduces myocardial ischemia/reperfusion injury. Stem Cell Research. 2010;**4**(3):214-222

[86] Bruno S et al. Microvesicles derived from mesenchymal stem cells enhance survival in a lethal model of acute kidney injury. PLoS One. 2012;**7**(3):e33115

[87] Hu GW et al. Exosomes secreted by human-induced pluripotent stem cell-derived mesenchymal stem cells attenuate limb ischemia by promoting angiogenesis in mice. Stem Cell Research & Therapy. 2015;**6**(1):1-15

[88] Conforti A et al. Microvesicles derived from mesenchymal stromal cells are not as effective as their cellular counterpart in the ability to modulate immune responses in vitro. Stem Cells and Development. 2014;**23**(21):2591-2599

[89] Di Trapani M et al. Differential and transferable modulatory effects of mesenchymal stromal cell-derived extracellular vesicles on T, B and NK cell functions. Scientific Reports. 2016;**6**:24120

[90] Del Fattore A et al. Immunoregulatory effects of mesenchymal stem cell-derived extracellular vesicles on T lymphocytes. Cell Transplantation. 2015;**24**(12):2615-2627

[91] Chen W et al. Immunomodulatory effects of mesenchymal stromal cells-derived exosome. Immunologic Research. 2016;**64**(4):831-840

[92] Zhang B, Yin Y, Lai RC, Tan SS, Choo ABH, Lim SK. Mesenchymal stem cells secrete immunologically active exosomes. Stem Cells and Development. 2013;**23**(11):1233-1244

[93] Blazquez R et al. Immunomodulatory potential of human adipose mesenchymal stem cells derived exosomes on in vitro stimulated T cells. Frontiers in Immunology. 2014;**5**(Nov):1-9

[94] Favaro E et al. Human mesenchymal stem cells and derived extracellular vesicles induce regulatory dendritic cells in type 1 diabetic patients. Diabetologia. 2016;**59**(2):325-333

[95] Bai L et al. Effects of mesenchymal stem cell-derived exosomes on experimental autoimmune uveitis. Scientific Reports. 2017;**7**:4323

[96] Kordelas L et al. MSC-derived exosomes: A novel tool to treat therapy-refractory graft-versus-host disease. Leukemia. 2014;**28**(4):970-973

[97] Quesenberry P, Levitt L. Hematopoietic stem cells. The New England Journal of Medicine. 1979;**301**(14):755-760

[98] Marbán E. The secret life of exosomes: What bees can teach us about next-generation therapeutics. Journal of the American College of Cardiology. 2018;**71**(2):193-200

[99] Levine JE, Paczesny S, Sarantopoulos S. Clinical applications for biomarkers of acute and chronic graft-versus-host disease. Biology of Blood and Marrow Transplantation. 2013;**18**:1-16

[100] Szyska M, Na I-K. Bone marrow GvHD after allogeneic hematopoietic stem cell transplantation. Frontiers in Immunology. 2016;7(March):1-6

[101] Griffin MD, Elliman SJ, Cahill E, English K, Ceredig R, Ritter T. Concise review: Adult mesenchymal stromal cell therapy for inflammatory diseases: How well are we joining the dots? Stem Cells. 2013;**31**(10):2033-2041

[102] Hedegaard CJ, Krakauer M, Bendtzen K, Lund H, Sellebjerg F, Nielsen CH. T helper cell type 1 (Th1), Th2 and Th17 responses to myelin basic protein and disease activity in multiple sclerosis. Immunology. 2008;**125**(2):161-169

[103] Melmed GY et al. Human placenta-derived cells (PDA-001) for the treatment of moderate-to-severe Crohn's disease: A phase 1b/2a study. Inflammatory Bowel Diseases. 2015;**21**(8):1809-1816

[104] Wang W et al. IL-37b gene transfer enhances the therapeutic efficacy of mesenchymal stromal cells in DSS-induced colitis mice. Acta Pharmacologica Sinica. 2015;**36**(11):1377-1387

[105] Tibboel J, Keijzer R, Reiss I, de Jongste JC, Post M. Intravenous and Intratracheal mesenchymal stromal cell injection in a mouse model of pulmonary emphysema. COPD. 2013;(416):131202132152003

[106] Bonfield TL, Koloze M, Lennon DP, Zuchowski B, Yang SE, Caplan AI. Human mesenchymal stem cells suppress chronic airway inflammation in the murine ovalbumin asthma model. American Journal of Physiology-Lung Cellular and Molecular Physiology. 2010;**299**(6):L760-L770

Chapter 7

Current State of the Art in DNA Vaccine Delivery and Molecular Adjuvants: Bcl-xL Anti-Apoptotic Protein as a Molecular Adjuvant

Sultan Gulce-Iz and Pelin Saglam-Metiner

Abstract

DNA vaccines (nucleic acid vaccines) have been gaining importance as promising therapeutics against infectious diseases, cancer, autoimmune disorders and allergy for the past two decades. However, the immune responses elicited by the DNA vaccines are not at the desired level to stimulate a protective immune response. Thus, studies are focused on the enhancement of DNA vaccine-induced immune response by different approaches. The most common approach is to use biomaterial-based adjuvants for enhanced antigen delivery and uptake by antigen-presenting cells. Some of these adjuvants are alum, saponins, microspheres, nanoparticles, liposomes, polymers, etc. used in vaccine formulations. In addition, molecular adjuvants like cytokines, chemokines and heat shock proteins have been shown to be promising in designing DNA vaccines. In this chapter, molecular adjuvants to improve DNA vaccination-induced immune responses will be summarized with a special focus on Bcl-xL anti-apoptotic protein.

Keywords: DNA vaccine, molecular adjuvant, delivery systems, antigen-presenting cells, Bcl-xL anti-apoptotic protein

1. DNA vaccine

DNA vaccine is a third-generation vaccine, which encompasses a vector with eukaryotic cell promoter, and a gene, which encodes for an immunogenic protein. These vaccines have been shown to elicit a robust cytotoxic T cell in comparison with subunit vaccines. Also, DNA vaccine has the capacity to induce both cellular and humoral immune responses by utilizing MHC I and MHC II antigen presentation by DCs [1–3]. Although DNA vaccines are licensed for use in veterinary vaccines since 2005, they have their own limitation due to low transfection efficiency. As a result, they perform poorly in human clinical trials and require multiple booster doses to achieve desirable immune response [2, 4, 5]. With the advent of new adjuvant systems such as nanoparticles, the immunogenicity of DNA vaccines can be enhanced considerably [1]. DNA vaccines are being currently used against a wide variety of infectious diseases as well as cancer [3].

1.1 Antigen presentation to T lymphocytes

Surface receptors of T lymphocytes interact with antigens to mount an immune response [6]. For the antigenic features; alienation, molecular weight, the delivery route to the organism is very important. At the molecular level, these receptors interact with the phagocyte cell or infected target cell, which carries antigen on its surface bound to the major histocompatibility complex (MHC). While T cells do not recognize natural antigens, antigens must first be processed by antigen-presenting cells (APCs) and then presented to the T cells with the relevant MHC protein. T cells (cytotoxic T cells—Tc) with CD8 (cluster of differentiation 8) receptors recognize MHC I antigens, while T cells (helper T cells—Th) with CD4 receptor recognize antigens on MHC II. Macrophages are the first identified antigen-presenting cells. Then, dendritic cells and B cells were identified. T-cell receptors (TCRs) are proteins that have spread through the membrane extending from the cell surface to the outer periphery. Each cell carries thousands of the same receptor surface. TCRs recognize and bind only bound peptide antigens on MHC [7, 8].

1.1.1 Major histocompatibility complex (MHC)

MHC proteins are encoded by the respective gene in the genome of all the vertebrate animals. The human MHC proteins are called human leukocyte antigens (HLAs) (human MHC I antigens, HLA-A, B and C, human MHC II antigens, HLA-DR, DQ and DP). Because of the difference in MHC proteins between the tissue donor and recipient, they were first discovered with tissue transplant rejection. Even within a species, these proteins are not structurally the same because of differences in amino acid sequences, also known as polymorphisms. For this reason, it forms an important antigenic barrier in organ transplantation. MHC genes encode two classes of MHC proteins, class I and class II. While MHC class I protein is located on the surfaces of all the nucleated cells, MHC class II protein is located only on the surface of antigen-presenting cells (APCs), including B lymphocytes, macrophages and dendritic cells. The structure of the MHC I protein comprises of a relatively small size of the β-2 microglobulin protein with α1, α2 and α3 domains linked to each other by disulfide bonds. The α1 and α2 domains constitute the variable antigen-binding domain. MHC II protein is formed by α1, β1, α2 and β2 domains, each of which is attached to one of the non-covalent bonds, and α1 and β1 domains constitute the antigen-binding domain, which is a variable part [7, 9, 10].

MHC proteins carry proteins in the cell which they are in, on themself. Thus, if the cell is not infected, it will carry its own peptides on the MHC proteins. On the other hand, if the cell harbors a foreign pathogen or protein, it will contain foreign peptides on MHC proteins. The function of these MHC proteins is to allow T cells to recognize foreign antigen. The T cells constantly control the surface of other cells for foreign antigen presence and do not recognize foreign antigens unless they are presented through MHC proteins. No T cell interacts with MHC on a healthy cell surface, and self-attacking cells are eliminated during the development of tolerance. During antigen presentation, the MHC and peptide complex come out of the cell membrane and thus are recognized by the T cells. There are two different antigen presentations to T cells, MHC I and MHC II antigen presentation [7–9].

1.1.2 Antigen presentation via MHC I protein

Peptides that are processed endogenously in the cytoplasm of non-phagocytic cells are presented with MHC I proteins. These antigens are derived from viruses or intracellular pathogens that infect cells, also known as internal antigens. In this pathway, for example, in a virus-infected cell, virus-associated proteins are primarily digested in the cytoplasmic proteasome. Peptide antigens of about 10 amino acids are delivered to the endoplasmic reticulum (ER), and a pore protein (TAP) produced by the two proteins acts in this stage. The peptides are bound to the MHC I protein, which results in the chaperone protein, which retains the MHC protein at that site. The resulting complex is released from the ER and goes to the cell surface and integrates into the membrane. This complex is recognized and bound by cytotoxic T cells. The CD8 receptor on the Tc cell surface strengthens it by adding the binding complex. This binding allows cytotoxic T cells to produce perforin and cytotoxic proteins that kill infected cells [7, 8, 10, 11].

1.1.3 Antigen presentation via MHC II protein

The MHC II protein is produced only in cells that present phagocytic antigen. For example, if an extracellular pathogen such as a bacterium is engulfed and then peptide antigens are provided, then MHC II proteins are produced in the ER and accumulated therein blocked with Li proteins, which inhibit binding with other peptides. The MHC II-Li protein complex is transferred to lysozyme and then combined with the phagosome to form the phagolysosome. There are foreign pathogen antigens, pathogenic proteins including connective chaperones are digested to form peptides of 10–15 amino acids. The resulting pathogenic peptides are transferred to the cell surface by binding with MHC II. This complex is recognized by the TCR on the helper T cells; the CD4 coreceptor also binds to this complex and, through interaction with the Th cells, activates to produce cytokines. The produced cytokine activates antibody production by specific B-cell clones or causes inflammation [7, 8, 11].

1.2 Advantages and disadvantages of DNA vaccination

The structure of plasmid DNA provides an advantage over other traditional protein-based or carbohydrate-based grafts in which it inherently possesses DNA vaccination. Immunogenesis from DNA vaccination takes a long time, and there is no pathogenicity caused by inactivated virus in DNA vaccines. The vaccine containing plasmid DNA (pDNA) can encode many immunogenic proteins of the same virus and can also encode similar proteins belonging to different infective agents [12]. Another important advantage is that the production of DNA vaccines is easier when compared to recombinant protein vaccines [13]. DNA vaccines prepared to make the cytokines more desirable to direct the immune system are more potent and suitable for stimulating the type of immunological response by cloning genes encoding the target cytokine and antigens into the same expression plasmids. DNA vaccines lead to sustained stimulation of antigen expression and the immune response leading to prolonged protective immunity [7]. Easy construction and manipulation of plasmid DNA are another important advantage of DNA vaccines [14].

DNA vaccines are stable at room temperature, are easy to obtain, are economical and are relatively more reliable than other vaccines. Plasmid DNA vaccines have been shown to be highly evaluated, safe and immunogenic in human clinical trials, even though they have no mental status [15]. However, it is necessary to increase transfection efficiencies of naked DNA vaccines, facilitate intracellular uptake, target into cells, and perform these operations with small amounts of DNA. Various gene delivery systems and adjuvant systems in the nanosphere are used to overcome these problems. During the use of nanotechnological adjuvant systems, the degradation of DNA is prevented, resulting in ultra-rapid delivery by targeting to desired cells [9, 16].

2. Delivery systems for DNA vaccine

2.1 Viral gene delivery systems

Viral-based gene delivery systems are carriers on which modifications are made to transfer therapeutic genes to target cells without creating viral disease. Viral gene carriers such as adenoviruses, adeno-associated viruses, lentiviruses and retroviruses exhibit an effective ability to transfer genetic material to the target cell with high gene transfer efficiency [17–19]. In viral gene delivery systems, the transferred genetic material either remains an episomal element or is integrated into the host chromosome. Desired genetic placement leads to persistent and stable protein expression but increases with the introduction of oncogenic potential mutagenesis [18, 20]. In addition, viral vectors being targeted to specific cell types, the limited availability of DNA, and the laborious and expensive large-scale production have led to a growing disincentive for the development of non-viral gene carriers. The safety risk is lower for non-viral carriers compared to viral gene carriers [18, 21–24].

2.2 Non-viral gene delivery systems

2.2.1 Physical delivery systems

Physical gene transfection delivery systems are consisting of Non-viral gene delivery systems are in which pDNA is usually applied alone, which involves mechanical processes such as microinjection, biojector, pressure and particle bombardment (gene gun), ultrasound, magnetofection, photoporation (laser assisted), hydroporation (hydrodynamic forced), droplet-based microfluidic platforms for in vitro transfection and electrical processes such as electroporation [10, 11, 21, 23, 25]. In addition, ultrasound and microbubble-mediated plasmid DNA uptake is a fast, global and multi-mechanisms involved process [26, 27].

2.2.1.1 Microinjection

In microinjection, cell membrane or nuclear membrane is penetrated by simple mechanical force using a microneedle diameter of 0.5–5 μm, at a specific and reproducible depth with less physical pain than conventional DNA delivery. This gene delivery system is mainly used to inject DNA constructs in vivo. Application of DNA by this method leads to constant expression of the antigen encoded in the skin. This method can also be used to deliver DNA for a prolonged period of time, similar to the administration of drugs at a constant rate. In the method, usually the stratum corneum and the viable epidermis are breached by microneedles, after which DNA can be delivered into the dermis. There are several different microneedle methods for DNA delivery; solid microneedles can be coated with DNA prior to skin penetration, uncoated microneedles can be used to damage the epidermis prior to application of a transdermal patch containing the DNA of interest, solid microneedles constructed with biopolymers can be coated with DNA such that the needles dissolve upon contact with the fluid in the dermis to release DNA into the skin and hollow microneedles can deliver DNA into the dermis through the needles [28–30]. Quantitative introduction of multiple components into the same cell is an advantage of this technique, while technical skills are required to prevent cell damage [31].

2.2.1.2 Gen gun

The ballistic DNA delivery or DNA-coated particle bombardment (gene gun) that was first used for gene transfer to plants in 1987 uses heavy metal microparticles (e.g., gold, silver microparticles or tungsten, 1–5 μm in diameter) to hold nucleic acids and penetrate the target cells. Momentum allows penetration of these particles to a few millimeters of the tissue and then cellular DNA release. Gas pressure, particle size and dose frequency are critical factors in determining the degree of tissue damage and penetration effectiveness of the application [18, 28]. This method has various advantages such as safety, high efficiency against parenteral injection, total amount of DNA required for delivery is low, no receptor is required, size of DNA is not a problem and production of DNA-coated metal particles is easy to generate. A major disadvantage is that it induces greater immune responses than microinjection due to tissue damage with intradermal delivery, even in low doses, and also, gene expression is short term and low. This technique is a widely tested method for intramuscular, intradermal and intratumoral genetic immunization. The use of gene gun for gene therapy against various cancers in clinical trials has also been demonstrated [18, 28–30].

2.2.1.3 Biojector

This device is commonly used to deliver medications through the skin for intradermal, subcutaneous and intramuscular applications. Usually, CO_2 pressure is used to force medications (e.g., vaccine) loaded in the device through a tiny orifice, which creates a high-pressure stream capable of penetrating the skin in the absence of a needle [28–30]. Biojectors have been used to deliver different kinds of vaccines such as DNA vaccine, in preclinical studies and human clinical trials to elicit significantly higher antibody responses and cell-mediated immunity (CMI) to the conventional (needle and syringe) vaccine delivery systems [29]. Because biojector-based delivery systems can increase the uptake of DNA in tissues of the skin and muscle, efficacy of the DNA vaccine is considerably increased. In a phase 1 trial for HIV vaccine, the success demonstrated with biojector used to enhance the efficiency of DNA transfection coupled with the fact that biojectors do not use needles that will most likely lead to the increased use of biojectors for DNA delivery in the clinic [28–30].

2.2.1.4 Electroporation

Electroporation was first studied on the degradation of cell membrane with electric induction in the 1960s. The first reported study is transfection of eukaryotic culture cells through electroporation in 1982 [18, 28]. In many subsequent studies, transfection was performed on animal and plant cells via electroporation [18]. This physical gene delivery technique uses electrical pulse to generate transient pores in the cell plasma membrane allowing efficient transfer of DNA into the cells. Pore formation occurs very rapidly, in approximately 10 ns. The size of the electric pore is estimated to be smaller than 10-nm radius. If the molecule is smaller than the pore size (as in oligonucleotides and chemical compounds), it can be transferred to the cell cytosol through diffusion [18, 28]. This method has been effectively applied in humans in order to enhance gene transfer and tested in several clinical trials such as prostate cancer [28, 30], leukemia [28], colorectal cancer [28], malignant melanoma [28, 30], brain carcinomas [28], Parkinson's disease [28], Alzheimer's disease [28] and depression [28]. When the parameters are optimized, this method is equally effective as viral vectors for in vivo application. But, the disadvantage is that it often results in a high incidence of cell death because of high temperature due to high voltage application. And also, transfection of the cells in large regions of the tissues is difficult [18, 28–30].

2.2.1.5 Ultrasound

Ultrasound (US) is a promising tool for gene delivery that has been able to facilitate DNA transfection of cells. US-mediated delivery is of interest due to its potential for repeated application, organ specificity, broad applicability to acoustically accessible organs, low toxicity and low immunogenicity. Different kinds of studies have examined gene transfection in various types of cells in vitro and with various organs and tissues in vivo, including brain [26, 30], cornea [30], pancreas [30], skeletal muscle [26, 30], liver [26, 30], heart [26, 30] and kidney [26, 30]. The advantages are that only acoustic energy is introduced into the cellular environment, which avoids possible safety concerns associated with chemical, viral or other materials introduced and left behind by other methods. Also, US-mediated delivery has been seen in many kinds of cell types and so may be broadly applicable, in contrast to other methods that often require reformulation for specific cell types. Unlike chemical delivery systems, US-mediated DNA uptake is often shown to be non-endocytotic. Acoustic cavitation plays a major role in the cell membrane permeabilization that facilitates DNA uptake. US can possibly deliver plasmid DNA to the periphery of the cell nucleus and facilitate rapid transfection by altering the cytoskeletal network. However, US-based gene transfection studies are still in preclinical trials and have the major challenge of relatively low transfection efficiency compared to optimal complexed chemical formulations and viral gene delivery systems [26, 28, 30].

The use of ultrasonication with the microbubble technique has shown great potential for intracellular gene delivery. The microbubble-cell membrane interaction serves as the key element bridging the acoustic conditions and the endpoint delivery outcomes. However, since the fundamental mechanical question of how plasmid DNA enters the intracellular space mediated by ultrasound and microbubbles is not fully understood, gene transfection efficiency is much lower than the potential for large-scale clinical needs [26, 27]. In one study, the gene transfection of human prostate cancer cell line (DU145) with fluorescently labeled DNA (pDNA gWiz-GFP) was studied after ultrasound exposure. In this process, different sonication conditions have been studied. DNA uptake, location of DNA during its intracellular trafficking and gene transfection efficiency after ultrasound exposure were followed for various periods by confocal microscopy and flow cytometry. As a result, ultrasounds delivered DNA into cell nuclei shortly after sonication and that the rest of the DNA cleared by autophagosomes/autophagolysosomes [26]. Also, ultrasound application combined with microbubbles has shown good potential for gene delivery. In one study, to unveil the detailed intracellular uptake process of plasmid DNA stimulated by ultrasound and microbubbles, the role of microbubbles in this process was investigated. So, targeted microbubbles were used to apply intracellular local stimulation on the cell membrane, and high-speed video microscopic recordings of microbubble dynamics were correlated with post-ultrasound 3D fluorescent confocal microscopic images fixed immediately after the cell. Two ultrasound conditions (high pressure, short pulse and low pressure, long pulse) were chosen to trigger different plasmid DNA uptake routes. Results showed that plasmid DNA uptake evoked by localized acoustically excited microbubbles was a fast (<2 min), global (not limited to the site where microbubbles were attached) and multi-mechanisms involved process [27].

2.2.2 Chemical adjuvant systems

The term adjuvant is derived from the Latin word "adjuvare" which means "help" or "develop." Adjuvants are used to increase the life, quality and degree of the specific immune response developed against the antigens. At the same time, they have low toxicity and are capable of sustaining the immunological activity alone by inhibiting polymer accumulation in the cell [11, 32, 33]. So, they are preferred in vaccinations for newborns or adults. Also, they can stimulate a long-term immune response by reducing the amount of antigen that must be given in a single dose of vaccine [9, 34].

Adjuvants are classified according to the source of their constituents, their physicochemical properties or their mechanism of action and are generally grouped into two subheadings. One of them is molecular adjuvants that are immunostimulants (and also genetic adjuvants) (e.g., TLR ligands, cytokines, saponins and bacterial exotoxins that stimulate the immune response) and act directly on the immune system to enhance immune response against antigens. The other one is carrier systems; they are systems that promote vaccine antigens in the most appropriate way to the immune system while also exhibiting controlled release and depot effects, thereby increasing the immune response (e.g., mineral salts, emulsions, liposomes, virosomes, biodegradable polymer micro/nano particles and immune stimulating complexes—ISCOMs) [1, 9, 11, 34–39].

Cytokines can also be delivered directly with the DNA vaccine, either on the same or on a separate expression plasmid as adjuvant duty. The effects of plasmid encoding cytokines such as interleukin IL-10, IL-12 or IFN-γ together with DNA vaccines have been studied in a variety of animal and disease models, up to clinical trials in humans [38]. Also, various studies describe the usage of plasmids coding for immune-signaling molecules, either as partial or as full-length genes. Many adjuvants function by activating the innate immune system via binding to Toll-like receptors (TLRs). Another innate immune mechanism, which is being explored for improving DNA vaccination, is the sensing of viral infections via pathogen recognition receptors (PRRs). Both proteins detect the presence of viral RNA in the cytosol. Co-delivery adjuvants with the vector coding for antigenic proteins result in significantly higher antibody titers as compared to the non-adjuvanted controls. Other strategies for genetic adjuvants include components of the complement system, protein aggregation domains, chemokines or co-stimulatory molecules. Whereas DNA vectors encoding certain cytokines have already entered clinical testing in humans, studies with many other genetic adjuvants were mostly performed in mice. Therefore, these promising studies should be optimized into powerful strategies to boost DNA vaccines in more complicated animals and humans [38].

Adjuvants can easily be internalized by the antigen-presenting cells (APCs) (macrophages and dendritic cells) because of their size being similar to pathogens (<10 μm) [11, 22, 25, 40]. The internalization and presentation of the adjuvant depends on the chemical and physical properties of the adjuvant system. It has been shown in various studies that the particles with cationic properties are more efficiently taken up by macrophages and dendritic cells [21, 24, 25, 41–43].

The characteristics that should be present in the adjuvants can be listed as follows: stability in an acidic, basic and enzymatic environment; retention of retained antigen or nucleic acid by constant release; systemic and mucosal immunity being effectively induced and balance between effective immunity and immunological tolerance at high doses [9, 44]. Also, the immunogenicity of weak antigens should increase the speed and duration of the immune response, cause only minimal local and systemic side effects, and be capable of a wide variety of vaccination with stability and ease of production. The ability to be effective in the living system of adjuvants depends on its ability to stimulate antigen-presenting cells (dendritic cells and macrophages) and T and B lymphocytes of the natural defense system [11]. There is a need for definitive information on the structure, stability, safety and immunogenicity of the adjuvant to be used in an effective vaccine development process [32, 33]. For this purpose, the choice of adjuvant depends on factors such as antigenic structure, immunization scheme, mode of administration and desired immune response pattern [33].

2.2.2.1 Nanoparticulate adjuvant systems and DNA vaccine delivery

Nanoparticles are matrix systems called nanospheres or nanocapsules according to the method of preparation, which vary in size from 1 to 1000 nm and are prepared with natural or synthetic materials. They are also the matrix systems in which the active substance nucleic acid is solubilized, adsorbed or electrostatically interacted with the surface [23, 45].

In vaccine development studies, nanotechnology is becoming increasingly important. Numerous nanoparticles of varying composition, size, shape and surface properties are used to both increase vaccine efficacy and target vaccination. With these properties, nanoparticles play an active role in in vitro/in vivo drug and gene delivery systems. Because nanoparticles are biodegradable and easily recognizable by antigen-presenting cells (APCs), they can be easily endocytosed and used as successful vaccine carriers in vaccine delivery systems [22, 25, 40].

Nanoparticle-mediated delivery of DNA vaccines has the advantages of increasing transfection efficiency and immunogenicity, inducing both cellular and antibody responses, and not requiring special equipment during administration; there are some disadvantages, such as, the long-term effects of nanoparticles in the body are not yet known [1]. As a DNA vaccine carrier, natural polymeric nanoparticles such as chitosan, alginate, pullulan and inulin (2–1000 nm); synthetic polymeric nanoparticles such as PLGA, dendrimer, PLA, PHB and PEI (2–1000 nm); inorganic nanoparticles such as gold, silica-based and carbon-based nanoparticles (2–1000 nm); nano-liposomes (100–400 nm) which are phospholipids that can be organized in nanoscale and non-infectious virus-like particles (VLP) (20–800 nm) generated by packaging the nucleic acid into biocompatible capsid proteins [1, 9, 22] are used. In recent years, the use of complex nanoparticles to overcome the disadvantages of enhancing the function of single-source nanoparticles has been discussed. Polyethylene/PLGA, polyg-glutamic acid/chitosan, polyethylene/chitosan, dendrimer/polyethylene glycol, polyg-glutamic acid/polyethyleneimine (PEI), chitosan/tripolyphosphate and polyethylene glycol/liposome nanoparticles are remarkable DNA transport systems [1, 22, 25, 40, 46, 47]. The overall efficiency of nanoparticle-based DNA delivery systems depends on four basic factors. These factors explain the necessity of nanoparticle-based adjuvant systems. Accurate plasmid DNA is integrated with the nanoparticle into the target cell correctly, the nanoparticle is removed from the endosomal vesicles and is transferred to the cytoplasm, then is transferred to the mitochondria or nucleus [23, 25].

In recent years, there has been a tremendous improvement in the area of gene delivery system with the advent of cationic polymers. These polymers bind with nucleic acid(s) to form complex structures known as polyplexes, which have increased transfection efficiency [10, 48]. Some of the examples of the polycationic polymers are chitosan, polyethyleneimine (PEI), poly(2-hydroxy ethyl methacrylate) (pHEMA), polyamidoamine (PAMAM) dendrimers, polylactic-co-glycolic acid (PLGA), polyethylene glycol (PEG) and poly-L-lysine (PLL) and the negatively charged phosphate group of pDNA, which have cationic properties. [10, 23, 42, 43, 49–51]. Many factors such as molecular weight (MW), surface charge, charge density, hydrophilicity and morphology significantly influence the gene transfection efficiency of cationic polymers. For this reason, in general, optimization of various forms of these cationic polymers with pDNA is required to increase transfection efficiency. The polyplex structure electrostatically formed with DNA packs it into smaller structure, pDNA, that interacts effectively with the negatively charged cell membrane and is endocytosed easily into the cell. In addition, cationic polymers are suitable for specific applications like conjugation of targeted ligands and various moieties, which provide them with specific characteristics [21, 22, 24, 25, 52].

2.2.2.1.1 Liposomes

Since their discovery in 1964, liposomes are extensively studied and used in the pharmaceutical and cosmetic industries. It is a generic name for single- or multi-lamellar vesicles in lipid-based nano- and micro-dimensions, whose surface charge can be changed by lipid formulation. Thanks to biocompatibility, biodegradability, low toxicity and low immunogenicity, liposomes have been used as potential nucleic acid carriers both in vitro and in vivo systems. In the composition of cationic liposomes, neutral lipids, cationic lipids and/or anionic lipids can be complexed in different ratios for creating ideal co-lipid. Neutral lipids (DOPE, DPPC, DOPC and Chol) are also often involved in the cationic liposome structure for more efficient transport systems, although sometimes only cationic lipids (DOTAP, DC-Chol, MMRIE, DODAP, DDTAP and DDA) are used [8, 36, 53]. The choice of ideal co-lipids is important during the formulation phase [54–56], since they significantly affect the overall performance of cationic liposomes.

There is a strong correlation between morphology and performance of lipoplex (liposome and DNA complex). There are several models that determine morphology such as the external model (DNA is attached to the cationic liposome surface), the internal model (DNA is surrounded by the cationic liposomes), the cationic liposome beads model on the DNA sequence and the spherical model. In addition to the liposomal composition, cationic lipid/nucleic acid (N/P) load ratio, preparation methods, ionic strength and temperature also affect lipoplex formulation and morphology. While high N/P ratios accept that the lipid/DNA complex is compatible with the global model with effective DNA concentration [22, 54, 57, 58], the low N/P ratio accepts the model of cationic liposome beads on the DNA sequence. In addition, high concentrations of cationic liposomes can cause cytotoxicity. The particle size of the lipoplexes is also influential on transfection efficiency. In general, large lipoplexes are more effective with in vitro transfection of nucleic acids because large pieces allow rapid sedimentation, maximum cell contact with the cell membrane and easier separation after endocytosis. Small particles, on the other hand, are much more effective, safe and suitable for in vivo transport of nucleic acids [57, 59].

Various studies have shown that cationic liposomes (DC-Chol/DOPE) formed at various ratios of 3β-[N-(N′,N′-dimethylaminoethane) carbamoyl] cholesterol (DC-Chol) and 1,2-dioleoyl-sn-glycero-3-phosphatidylethanolamine (DOPE) are effective pDNA carriers in the preclinical as well clinical trials for plasmid transfection [55, 57, 60]. In another study, it was reported that the vaccine adjuvants with high immunogenicity were obtained with cationic liposomes formed at 50:50 ratio (50 mol%) with DC-Chol/DPPC (3β-[N-(N′,N′-dimethylaminoethane) carbamoyl] cholesterol/1,2-dipalmitoyl-sn-glycero-3-phosphocholine) [53]. In many studies, it has been reported that surface modifications to cationic liposomes (PEG-polyethylene glycol coating, etc.) increase transfection efficiency due to more stable plasmid retention, longer circulation time and lower immunological response. Studies have shown that transfection efficiency is increased by about 55% with PEG coating to protect surface charges [23, 48, 54, 56, 57, 61].

2.2.2.1.2 Chitosan

Chitosan is the best-known working polymer among the therapeutic natural polymers. It consists of D-glucosamine and N-acetyl-D-glucosamine units linked by β-(1,4) glycosidic bonds. The chitosan is derived from the chitin molecule and the thermoacetal deacetylation process forms the bonds. The chitin is a biopolymer in abundance in nature and is the cell wall of most of the fungi and bacteria of the shellfish and the outer shell of insects [62]. One of the most important applications of chitosan is its application as non-viral vector in gene therapy. For this reason, chitosan has recently been used for gene delivery systems for therapeutic purposes [50, 63]. The first chitosan/DNA complex was made about 25 years ago, and was composed of plasmid and chitosan in size of 150–600 nm. Positive charge, which allows it to complex easily with negatively charged DNA, allows the formation of nanocapsules (80–500) at various sizes that protect DNA from nuclease activation [64, 65].

Chitosan nanoparticles are formed by a wide variety of methods, by the formation of different bonds, by different polymer conformations and by various internal and external molecular interactions. In addition to covalent cross-linking and desolvation methods, ionic gelation is one of the most useful methods used in the handling of chitosan nanoparticles and is especially considered for polyelectrolyte sodium tripolyphosphate (TPP) [42, 43, 66]. In chitosan-based adjuvants, DNA is involved in structure determination, electrostatic interaction, encapsulation and surface adsorption [42, 50]. Chitosan has excellent biocompatibility, acceptable biodegradability, high biosecurity, low cytotoxicity and low immunogenicity. However, limited application of gene transport due to poor solubility at physiological pH, insufficient positive charge and low transfection efficiency can be prevented by various surface modifications on chitosan nanoparticles [25]. For example, TPP is useful in preparing chitosan nanoparticles and enhances its non-toxic nature. Due to the self-regulation nature of polycations and polyanions, it leads to the formation of linking complexes between TPP groups and chitosan amino groups. In the process of the protonation of the chitosan at physiological pH, TPP is covalently bound to chitosan amino groups providing structural change and better provocation [23, 50, 61, 67, 68].

2.2.2.1.3 Polyethyleneimine (PEI)

Polyethyleneimine is a gene-carrying cationic polymer that has high transfection efficiency in vitro and in vivo with lower cost, but can exhibit high toxicity with concentration pulse [69–71]. PEI receives proton in aqueous solutions and has a high positive charge. Thus, in vitro and in vivo DNA and oligonucleotide transport are promising candidates as non-viral transport systems [71, 72]. PEI and its derivatives are commonly known as an effective dispersant and cationic flocculent used for negatively charged colloids [73].

Adjuvant systems with PEI involve the electrostatic interaction of DNA with the cationic polymer and the formation of the polycation/DNA complex [74]. The DNA/polymer complex (N/P) occurs when the amine group of this polymer interacts with the phosphate group of DNA [73]. In many studies, it has been shown that PEI has the advantages of holding pDNA with electrostatic bonds, binding to the cell surface and its endocytosis, and releasing pDNA into the cell. It also enhances the entry of the gene from cytoplasm to the nucleus [70]. This polymer is used for DNA-based immunotherapy or DNA vaccine delivery to ensure that the immune response is activated to provide a strong immune response [74]. Factors such as molecular weight, branching grade, ionic strength of solution, zeta potential and particle size affect the efficacy/cytotoxicity of PEI. PEI is coated with PEG and various ligands to increase transfection efficiency and reduce cytotoxicity. Meanwhile, the PEI in the linear structure helps to create an effective transport system than the branched PEI [69].

2.2.2.1.4 Dendrimers

Dendrimers are nanometer-sized (1–100 nm) particles with a unique architectural structure in the form of spherical macromolecules, consisting of a central core, a hyperbranched mantle and a corona containing a peripheral reactive group. Dendrimers can be fabricated by convergent or divergent synthesis. The high-level control system on dendritic architectural synthesis makes dendrimers almost perfect spherical nanostructures with predictable properties. Dendrimers can build up ionic interactions with DNA, creating complexes with high stability and resolution. Costly production is the only disadvantage. Structures such as polyamidoamine and polypropylenimine are included in the dendrimeric classification [25, 75–78].

Of the cationic compounds used in gene delivery, polyamidoamine (PAMAM) dendrimers have been regarded as the most suitable gene carrier, due to the presence of abundant amino groups on the electrostatically interacting surface with negatively charged nucleic acid material and low polydispersity. This association at the nanoscale (nucleic acid-dendrimer pair) is called dendriplex [79]. These particular supramolecular structures not only protect the genetic material from nuclease degradation but also interact with the negative surface of the cell membrane and activate entry into the cell through endocytosis. The high amine content of PAMAM dendrimers provides significant buffering capacity in the endosomal pH range. This extraordinary buffering capacity plays a powerful driving force in the liberation of dendriplex complexes prior to enzymatic degradation to lysosomal enzymes in endosomes. These properties make PAMAM dendrimers the carriers that are obliged to carry out future polycation-based gene delivery studies. On the other hand, long-term storage stability and high biocompatibility make PAMAM dendrimers almost necessary to use as gene carriers in vivo [24, 25, 49, 51, 61, 75].

The number of generations on the transfection efficiency is important. Dendrimer generations G0–G3, low-grade PAMAM dendrimers, exhibit low gene transfection efficiency and low cytotoxicity, while G4–G8 dendrimers show high transfection efficiency and high cytotoxicity. For this reason, dendrimer generations G4–G5, which have low cytotoxicity as well as high transfection efficiency in gene transfer, are preferred [25, 76]. In addition, adding different moieties enhances various features of dendrimers. For example, high amine content on the PAMAM surface allows conjugation of various materials to improve transfection efficiency and reduce target cytotoxicity [24, 25, 49, 61]. PEG conjugation provides positively charged protective sheath, which reduces cytotoxicity, undesired interactions with blood components, and facilitates binding of the ligand. Adding hydrophobic moieties favors hydrophilic-hydrophobic balance, reduced cytotoxicity and facilitation of packaging back into the vector. With glucocorticoid conjugation, nuclear targeting and parental dendrimers (dexamethasone and triamcinolone acetonide conjugates) provide hydrophilic-hydrophobic equilibrium modulation. By cyclodextrin conjugation, increase of endosomal escape and decrease of cytotoxicity as well as oligonucleotides against enzymatic digestion are protected. Finally, by amino acid, peptide and protein conjugation, it is also possible to increase cell penetration (arginine and TAT peptide conjugation), cellular uptake, endosomal escape, serum resistance (histidine conjugation), and nuclear localization, and also target specific receptors [24, 25, 51, 61, 77, 78].

2.2.2.1.5 Poly(lactic-co-glycolic acid) (PLGA)

PLGA is a solid polymeric material approved by the Food and Drug Administration (FDA) for nanoparticle-based drug and gene delivery systems. Their biocompatibility, biodegradability, reliability and high stability characteristics during storage provide advantages in delivery systems [20, 80–82]. PLGA nanoparticles can easily pass through vessels in vivo without damaging the tissues surrounding the tumor and thus accumulate with the mechanism of “enhanced permeability retention” (EPR) in solid tumors. However, PLGA particles are less efficient in encapsulating nucleic acids because hydrophobic properties of PLGA are not compatible with anionic, hydrophilic properties of nucleic acids. In addition, difficult preparation conditions and pH decreases during PLGA hydrolysis inactivate nucleic acid loading and prevent polyplex formation. In order to overcome these drawbacks, effective gene transfer systems can be formed with different formulations made with different molecular interactions [21, 48, 52, 61, 83–86].

For example, PLGA nanoparticles can be processed with materials such as PEI to increase positive charge distribution and provide a stronger penetration of nucleic acid. After penetration of the nucleic acids, PEI, PEG cross-linking material and cell penetration peptides can be used for effective encapsulation and stabilization of the nano-carrier system [48, 81, 85]. It is also one of the systems to produce PLGA-based adjuvants in sizes of 200–300 nm by such means as cationic hydrophilic properties by condensing PLGA with cationic polymers such as polyethylenoxide (PEO) and polyethylene glycol methacrylate (PEGMA), emulsifying solvent diffusion method without shear stress [48, 81, 85].

In one study, DNA-loaded PLGA particles were fabricated by a double emulsion water in oil in water (w/o/w) method, in which energy is introduced to the system typically by either sonication or homogenization, and they were provided with submicron size (generally 0.1–10 μm). Then, conjugation of PLL to PLGA was achieved through the coupling agent at different percentages to create pDNA/PLGA/PLL (poly-l-lysine) complex. This system achieved effective gene transport by acquiring cationic adjuvant property. [87]. In another study, it has been reported that the PLGA particle, which is condensed with the cationic lipid DOTAP, provides efficient pDNA encapsulation by forming a cationic adjuvant system [88].

2.2.2.1.6 Polyethylene glycol (PEG)

Polyethylene glycol (PEG) is a highly hydrophilic, non-immunogenic, semicrystalline, linear polyether diol used as a non-ionic polymer consisting of ethylene oxide monomers. PEG, a polymer approved by the Food and Drug Administration (FDA), is non-toxic at low density and does not damage active proteins or cells. PEG is excreted completely through the kidneys (<30 kDa PEGs) or stool (>20 kDa PEGs) [89]. In addition, functionalities by conjugation of different terminal groups such as amino, carboxyl and sulfhydryl groups can be increased. It is soluble in aqueous solutions and in most organic solvents like methanol and dichloromethane [89].

The physical properties of the PEG material vary with the molecular weight. With an increase in the molecular weight, viscosity of PEG increases, while the water solubility decreases. Furthermore, the high solubility of PEG in organic solvents provides a great advantage in preparing solid dispersions. PEG provides stability to coating particles. The flexibility of the polymer chain, which allows the polymer units to rotate freely, ensures that the PEG protects the particles. Thanks to its high hydrophilic property, it creates a protective shield around the particulate. Nowadays, PEG is used not only to increase stability and circulation time of particles in vivo, but also to target particles to the desired areas [90].

In vivo transfection experiments with DC-Chol/DOPE liposomes with 1% PEG coating showed that the PEG coating increases the stability and longevity of the adjuvant, while it decreases the pH sensitivity and thus decreases the transfection rate. This pH sensitivity is important for the vaccination strategies carried out in the treatment of an existing tumor tissue [55]. However, there is no indirect disadvantage of PEG coating on the transfection rate, as there is no intention to improve the present tumor tissue, but there is no need for pH sensitivities for adjuvants in vaccine studies designed to protect against tumor formation [23, 54, 56, 61].

2.2.2.1.7 Poly(2-hydroxyethyl methacrylate) (pHEMA)

The pHEMA [poly(2-hydroxyethyl methacrylate)] polymer is the polymerized non-toxic form of HEMA (hydroxyethyl methacrylate) which is a toxic monomer. Hydrogels are hydrophilic and are capable of holding water up to thousands of times more than their own dry mass. For this purpose, pHEMA that is virtually uncharged is a three-dimensional hydrophobic polymer that can swell in water or biological fluids, and it can be used with a large number of pathways [91, 92]. Because of its high water content such as those in body cells, it is used in ureters, cardiovascular implants, contact lenses, tissue restorative surgical materials and many dental applications [93, 94]. pHEMA is also used in the pharmaceutical industry and in tissue engineering because of its biocompatibility and similar physical properties as living tissues [93]. In addition, the pHEMA polymer has been developed by virtue of its high biocompatibility properties and successful complexes formed by a wide variety of cationic compounds. It is also used in DNA purification, RNA adsorption and drug and enzyme transport [91, 95, 96]. These approaches shed light on the creation of new adjuvant systems for the transport of genetic material using pHEMA [91, 93, 97].

In our previous studies, we purposed to develop new pHEMA-based adjuvant systems to increase the immune effectiveness and protectivity of the DNA vaccine. Within this scope, cationic pHEMA-His/PEG, pHEMA-Chitosan/PEG, pHEMA-PEI/PEG and pHEMA-DOTAP/PEG particles were developed. As a result, all pHEMA-based adjuvant systems, which can be produced in nano-sizes and in the desired properties, have been shown to increase in vitro transfection efficiency compared to naked DNA by using them in different pDNA/adjuvant formulation ratios. When compared to Lipofectamine 2000 agent, pHEMA-PEI and pHEMA-DOTAP adjuvant formulations are promising candidates for gene transfection agents [98].

2.2.2.2 Characterization of adjuvant systems

Advances in adjuvant systems have led to the development of biodegradable, environmentally responsive and biocompatible vaccine carriers (e.g., droplet-based microfluidic devices). An ideal adjuvant system should effectively interact with both the pDNA and cellular membrane and should not elicit an immune response or cytotoxicity. Characterization studies of pDNA vaccine-loaded delivery systems are carried out by size and zeta potential measurements, transmission electron microscopy (TEM), scanning electron microscopy (SEM), atomic force microscopy (AFM), gel retardation assay with agarose gel electrophoresis, PicoGreen assays, robustness assays and FT-IR [26, 31, 99–102].

2.3 Cellular uptake of delivery systems

Cellular uptake adjuvant/nucleic acid formulations mainly depend on type, size, shape as well as composition, surface chemistry and/or the carrier charge. These are key factors, which affect carrier/cell interactions and the transfection efficiency. Cellular uptake of nucleic acid-loaded delivery systems and their localization in 2D (monolayer culture) and 3D (multicellular tumor spheroids) in vitro cell culture models and also in vivo models are studied by multi-labeling 3D confocal fluorescence microscopy, flow cytometry, overlaid bright field fluorescence microscopy based on GFP expressions, luciferase assays and fluorescence images [26, 27, 100–102].

3. Molecular adjuvants and Bcl-xL anti-apoptotic protein

Molecular adjuvants can be defined as plasmids expressing cytokines, chemokines or co-stimulatory molecules which can be co-administered with the antigenic DNA vaccine plasmid [103] or vaccine plasmid can be constructed as a bicistronic vector system. The magnitude of immune response after DNA vaccination is very closely related to: (i) the source of Ag presentation, (ii) the immunological properties of the DNA itself and (iii) the role of cytokines in eliciting the immune responses [104]. Thus, with the cells transfected by molecular adjuvant, encoding plasmids secrete the adjuvant into the surrounding region stimulating both local antigen-presenting cells (APCs) and cells in the draining lymph node, especially dendritic cells. The examples of molecular adjuvants as cytokines: GM-CSF (granulocyte-macrophage colony stimulating factor), M-CSF, IFN-γ, IL-2, IL-4, IL-7 and IL-8, IL-10, IL-12, IL-15, IL-18; as chemokines: IL-8, MCP-1 (monocyte chemoattractant protein 1), MIP-1a (macrophage inflammatory protein), RANTES (CCL5); and as co-stimulatory proteins: CD40L, CD80/86, ICAM-1 (intercellular adhesion molecule 1) [103]. In addition, ligands of pattern recognition receptors (PRRs) are described as molecular adjuvants. There are 13 TLR genes (TLR1–TLR13). TLR3 and TLR9 recognize dsRNA and ssDNA, respectively, and their ligands have been shown to act as molecular adjuvants. Poly(I:C) is a classical TLR3 ligand, and CpG is a TLR 9 ligand, showing molecular adjuvant properties via increasing cytotoxic T-cell responses [105]. Bcl-xL anti-apoptotic protein was also described as molecular adjuvant. Inhibiting the apoptosis of antigen-presenting dendritic cells, the cytotoxic T-cell responses (CD8+ T cells) are increased due to the longer survival of the dendritic cells [106]. In addition, rather than co-transfection, expression of Bcl-xL in a bicistronic vector further enhances CD8+ T-cell responses compared to co-transfection [107, 108].

In our previous studies, pIRESEGFP/Bcl-xL is a bicistronic vector bearing CMV (cytomegalovirus) promoter and IRES (internal ribosomal entry site) used as a backbone for DNA vaccination studies. Bcl-xL anti-apoptotic protein in frame with eGFP (enhanced green florescence protein) as a molecular adjuvant was also encoded by the plasmid. It's shown that Bcl-xL anti-apoptotic protein rescued cells from serum deprivation, doxorubicin, camptothecin and staurosporine induced apoptosis [71, 109], induced prolonged expression of the antigen of interest in expressed under CMV promoter that facilitates an increased CD8+ T cell response in DNA vaccination studies encoding foot and mouth disease multi-epitopes [4] and Toxoplasma gondii, SporoSAG antigen [5].

4. Conclusion

In this chapter, we have discussed DNA vaccines, several widely used and emerging gene delivery systems to increase efficacy of DNA vaccines, characterization of these systems and cellular uptake of DNA vaccines yet to be tested in the clinic in the future. Also, as means of molecular adjuvants, several agents are in consideration like chemokines, cytokines, co-stimulatory molecules, PPR ligands and anti-apoptotic proteins.

Nanotechnology offers new strategies in formulating better adjuvants for DNA vaccines. However, they are very stable and the long-term cytotoxic effects in the body appear to be a potential problem. In order to remove this problem, most effective surface and content modifications of nanoparticles studied are being made. The relatively short history of the use of nanoparticles has led to a lack of understanding of the safety profile of human use. For this reason, many studies are being carried out in this regard today. If a safe profile can be shown as a result of these studies, this new vaccine delivery system will be considered to be an effective method, which will be widely used. In addition, nanoparticle-based DNA vaccines are seen as a strategy for future single-dose applications and the need for needle-free vaccines, as they enhance cell transfection efficiency and immunogenicity and enable targeting strategies.

In future studies, the development of nanoparticle-based gene delivery systems for different purposes will continue to be critical. Modification of toxicity and immunogenicity problems of viral vectors, enhancement of transfection efficiency as much as possible for non-viral vectors, enhancement of vector targeting and specificity, regulation of gene expression and identification of synergies between gene-based agents and other cancer therapies are promising studies. Nevertheless, the safe and efficient transport of plasmid DNA to initiate immunological responses remains an important barrier to human DNA vaccination. The development of new non-viral strategies for DNA vaccines has to continue to serve as biological insight and clinic-related methods. Specific concerns include difficulties with transfection of dendritic cells. This includes methods that target strong antigen signaling, antigen-presenting cell uptake and lymph node transduction without sacrificing biocompatibility. Carriers must deliver the genetic load specifically to the target tissue, while protecting the genetic material from metabolic and immune pathways.

DNA transfection of cells in vitro/in vivo studies requires overcoming both extracellular and intracellular barriers to gene transport from cell plasma membrane which is the barrier of intracellular DNA uptake and hinders DNA trafficking in the cytoplasm, and also into the cell nucleus that is nuclear envelope. Therefore, gene delivery methods including viral, non-viral, physical, chemical and molecular systems should facilitate DNA delivery across these barriers and into the nucleus to enable transcription without any degradation very quickly. Gene delivery systems are so important that besides the characterization of these systems by various methods such as SEM, TEM, AFM and FT-IR, the examination of their cellular uptake by various techniques like confocal complex fluorescence microscopy and flow cytometry and the development of study done in this area are extremely important in the future.

Author details

Sultan Gulce-Iz[1,2,3]* and Pelin Saglam-Metiner[2]

1 Department of Bioengineering, Faculty of Engineering, Ege University, Izmir, Turkey

2 Bioengineering Graduate Programme, Institute of Natural and Applied Sciences, Ege University, Izmir, Turkey

3 Biomedical Technologies Graduate Programme, Institute of Natural and Applied Sciences, Ege University, Izmir, Turkey

*Address all correspondence to: sultangulce@gmail.com

References

[1] Gregory AE, Titball R, Williamson D. Vaccine delivery using nanoparticles. Frontiers in Cellular and Infection Microbiology. 2013. DOI: 10.3389/fcimb.2013.00013

[2] Silveira MM, Oliveira TL, Schuch RA, McBride AJA, Dellagostin OA, Hartwig DD. DNA vaccines against leptospirosis: A literature review. Vaccine. 2017. DOI: 10.1016/j.vaccine.2017.08.067

[3] Zahm CD, Colluru VT, McNeel DG. DNA vaccines for prostate cancer. Pharmacology & Therapeutics. 2017. DOI: 10.1016/j.pharmthera.2017.02.016

[4] Gülçe Iz S, Döşkaya M, Borrego B, Rodriguez F, Gürüz Y, Gürhan ID. Co-expression of the Bcl-xL antiapoptotic protein enhances the induction of Th1-like immune responses in mice immunized with DNA vaccines encoding FMDV B and T cell epitopes. Veterinary Research Communications. 2013. DOI: 10.1007/s11259-013-9560-3

[5] Gülçe Iz S, Döşkaya M, Caner A, Döşkaya AD, Rodriguez F, Gürüz Y, et al. A novel dual promoter DNA vaccine induces CD8+ response against toxoplasma gondii sporozoite specific surface protein "sporoSAG" through non-apoptotic cells. Trials in Vaccinology. 2014. DOI: 10.1016/j.trivac.2014.04.003

[6] Efe İris FN. Antijen ve Antijen Sunumu. Turkiye Klinikleri Journal of Infectious Diseases Special Topics. 2008;**1**:14-18

[7] Tüting T, Austyn J, Storkus WJ, Falo LD. The immunology of DNA vaccines. In: Lowrie DB, Whalen RG, editors. DNA Vaccines: Methods and Protocols. Totowa, New Jersey: Humana Press Inc; 2000. pp. 37-64. DOI: 10.1385/1592596886

[8] Morse MA, CLAY TM, Lyerly HK. Handbook of Cancer Vaccines. Totowa, New Jersey: Humana Press; 2004

[9] Hackett CJ, Harn DA, editors. Vaccine Adjuvants Immunological and Clinical Principles. Totowa, New Jersey: Humana Press; 2006

[10] Saltzman WM, Shen H, Brandsma JL. DNA Vaccines: Methods and Protocols. 2nd ed. In: Hackworth J, editor. Totowa, New Jersey: Humana Press Inc; 2006. DOI: 10.1385/1597451681

[11] Singh M, editor. Vaccine Adjuvants and Delivery Systems. Emeryville, California, United States of America: John Wiley; 2007

[12] Rajčáni J, Moško T, Režuchová I. Current developments in viral DNA vaccines: Shall they solve the unsolved? Reviews in Medical Virology. 2005. DOI: 10.1002/rmv.467

[13] Smooker PM, Rainczuk A, Kennedy N, Spithill TW. DNA vaccines and their application against parasites—Promise, limitations and potential solutions. Biotechnology Annual Review. 2004. DOI: 10.1016/S1387-2656(04)10007-0

[14] Colluru VT, Johnson LE, Olson BM, McNeel DG. Preclinical and clinical development of DNA vaccines for prostate cancer. Urologic Oncology: Seminars and Original Investigations. 2016. DOI: 10.1016/j.urolonc.2013.09.014

[15] Ulmer JB, Geall AJ. Recent innovations in mRNA vaccines. Current Opinion in Immunology. 2016. DOI: 10.1016/j.coi.2016.05.008

[16] Oster CG, Kim N, Grode L, Barbu-Tudoran L, Schaper AK, Kaufmann SHE, et al. Cationic microparticles consisting of poly(lactide-co-glycolide)

and polyethylenimine as carriers systems for parental DNA vaccination. Journal of Controlled Release. 2005. DOI: 10.1016/j.jconrel.2005.02.004

[17] Malboeuf CM, Simon DAL, Lee YEE, Lankes HA, Dewhurst S, Frelinger JG, et al. Human papillomavirus-like particles mediate functional delivery of plasmid DNA to antigen presenting cells in vivo. Vaccine. 2007. DOI: 10.1016/j.vaccine.2007.01.067

[18] Cevher E, Sezer AD, Çağlar EŞ. Gene delivery systems: Recent progress in viral and non-viral therapy. In: Sezer AD, editor. Recent Advances in Novel Drug Carrier Systems. London, UK: IntechOpen Science; 2012. pp. 437-470. DOI: 10.5772/2889

[19] Vandermeulen G, Athanasopoulos T, Trundley A, Foster K, Préat V, Yáñez-Muñoz RJ, et al. Highly potent delivery method of gp160 envelope vaccine combining lentivirus-like particles and DNA electrotransfer. Journal of Controlled Release. 2012. DOI: 10.1016/j.jconrel.2012.01.035

[20] Scheerlinck JPY, Greenwood DLV. Virus-sized vaccine delivery systems. Drug Discovery Today. 2008. DOI: 10.1016/j.drudis.2008.06.016

[21] Luo D, Saltzman WM. Synthetic DNA delivery systems. Nature Biotechnology. 2000. DOI: 10.1038/71889

[22] Zhao L, Seth A, Wibowo N, Zhao CX, Mitter N, Yu C, et al. Nanoparticle vaccines. Vaccine. 2014. DOI: 10.1016/j.vaccine.2013.11.069

[23] Adijanto J, Naash MI. Nanoparticle-based technologies for retinal gene therapy. European Journal of Pharmaceutics and Biopharmaceutics. 2015. DOI: 10.1016/j.ejpb.2014.12.028

[24] Dehshahri A, Sadeghpour H. Surface decorations of poly(amidoamine) dendrimer by various pendant moieties for improved delivery of nucleic acid materials. Colloids Surfaces B Biointerfaces. 2015. DOI: 10.1016/j.colsurfb.2015.05.006

[25] Jin L, Zeng X, Liu M, Deng Y, He N. Current progress in gene delivery technology based on chemical methods and nano-carriers. Theranostics. 2014. DOI: 10.7150/thno.6914

[26] Liu Y, Yan J, Santangelo PJ, Prausnitz MR. DNA uptake, intracellular trafficking and gene transfection after ultrasound exposure. Journal of Controlled Release. 2016. DOI: 10.1016/j.jconrel.2016.05.013

[27] Rong N, Zhou H, Liu R, Wang Y, Fan Z. Ultrasound and microbubble mediated plasmid DNA uptake: A fast, global and multi-mechanisms involved process. Journal of Controlled Release. 2018. DOI: 10.1016/j.jconrel.2018.01.014

[28] Agi E, Mosaferi Z, Khatamsaz S, Cheraghi P, Samadian N, Bolhassani A. Different strategies of gene delivery for treatment of cancer and other disorders. Journal of Solid Tumors. 2016;**6**:76-84. DOI: 10.5430/jst.v6n2p76

[29] Jorritsma SHT, Gowans EJ, Grubor-Bauk B, Wijesundara DK. Delivery methods to increase cellular uptake and immunogenicity of DNA vaccines. Vaccine. 2016. DOI: 10.1016/j.vaccine.2016.09.062

[30] Kamimura K, Suda T, Zhang G, Liu D. Advances in gene delivery systems. Pharmaceutical Medicine. 2011. DOI: 10.2165/11594020-000000000-00000

[31] Vitor MT, Sipoli CC, De La Torre LG. Droplet-based microfluidic systems for production and transfection in vitro of non-viral vectors for gene delivery. Research & Reviews: Journal of Pharmacy and Pharmaceutical Sciences. 2015

[32] Zou W, Liu C, Chen Z, Zhang N. Preparation and characterization of

cationic PLA-PEG nanoparticles for delivery of plasmid DNA. Nanoscale Research Letters. 2009. DOI: 10.1007/s11671-009-9345-3

[33] Badiee A, Heravi Shargh V, Khamesipour A, Jaafari MR. Micro/nanoparticle adjuvants for antileishmanial vaccines: Present and future trends. Vaccine. 2013. DOI: 10.1016/j.vaccine.2012.11.068

[34] Reed SG, Orr MT, Fox CB. Key roles of adjuvants in modern vaccines. Nature Medicine. 2013. DOI: 10.1038/nm.3409

[35] Harandi AM, Davies G, Olesen OF. Vaccine adjuvants: Scientific challenges and strategic initiatives. Expert Review of Vaccines. 2009. DOI: 10.1586/14760584.8.3.293

[36] Davies G, editor. Vaccine Adjuvants, Methods and Protocols. United Kingdom, London: Humana Press; 2010. DOI: 10.1007/978-1-60761-585-9

[37] Brito LA, O'Hagan DT. Designing and building the next generation of improved vaccine adjuvants. Journal of Controlled Release. 2014. DOI: 10.1016/j.jconrel.2014.06.027

[38] Grunwald T, Ulbert S. Improvement of DNA vaccination by adjuvants and sophisticated delivery devices: Vaccine-platforms for the battle against infectious diseases. Clinical and Experimental Vaccine Research. 2015. DOI: 10.7774/cevr.2015.4.1.1

[39] Rathbone M, Senel S, Pather I, editors. Oral mucosal drug delivery and therapy. In: Advances in Delivery Science and Technology. Boston, MA: Springer; 2015. DOI: 110.1007/978-1-4899-7558-4

[40] Treuel L, Jiang X, Nienhaus GU. New views on cellular uptake and trafficking of manufactured nanoparticles. Journal of the Royal Society Interface. 2013. DOI: 10.1098/rsif.2012.0939

[41] Felgner PL. Nonviral strategies for gene therapy. Scientific American. 1997. DOI: 10.1038/scientificamerican0697-102

[42] Mao S, Sun W, Kissel T. Chitosan-based formulations for delivery of DNA and siRNA. Advanced Drug Delivery Reviews. 2010. DOI: 10.1016/j.addr.2009.08.004

[43] Gaspar VM, Correia IJ, Sousa Â, Silva F, Paquete CM, Queiroz JA, et al. Nanoparticle mediated delivery of pure P53 supercoiled plasmid DNA for gene therapy. Journal of Controlled Release. 2011. DOI: 10.1016/j.jconrel.2011.08.007

[44] Xia Y, Fan Q, Hao D, Wu J, Ma G, Su Z. Chitosan-based mucosal adjuvants: Sunrise on the ocean. Vaccine. 2015. DOI: 10.1016/j.vaccine.2015.07.101

[45] Derman S, Kizilbey K, Akdeste MZ. Polimerik nanopartiküller. Sigma Journal of Engineering and Natural Sciences. 2013;**31**:107-120

[46] Minigo G, Scholzen A, Tang CK, Hanley JC, Kalkanidis M, Pietersz GA, et al. Poly-l-lysine-coated nanoparticles: A potent delivery system to enhance DNA vaccine efficacy. Vaccine. 2007. DOI: 10.1016/j.vaccine.2006.09.086

[47] Yameen B, Il CW, Vilos C, Swami A, Shi J, Farokhzad OC. Insight into nanoparticle cellular uptake and intracellular targeting. Journal of Controlled Release. 2014. DOI: 10.1016/j.jconrel.2014.06.038

[48] Bolhassani A, Javanzad S, Saleh T, Hashemi M, Aghasadeghi MR, Sadat SM. Polymeric nanoparticles: Potent vectors for vaccine delivery targeting cancer and infectious diseases. Human Vaccines & Immunotherapeutics. 2014. DOI: 10.4161/hv.26796

[49] Ke W, Shao K, Huang R, Han L, Liu Y, Li J, et al. Gene delivery targeted to the brain using an Angiopep-conjugated polyethyleneglycol-modified polyamidoamine dendrimer. Biomaterials. 2009. DOI: 10.1016/j.biomaterials.2009.08.049

[50] Carrillo C, Suñé JM, Pérez-Lozano P, García-Montoya E, Sarrate R, Fàbregas A, et al. Chitosan nanoparticles as non-viral gene delivery systems: Determination of loading efficiency. Biomedicine & Pharmacotherapy. 2014. DOI: 10.1016/j.biopha.2014.07.009

[51] Wang Y, Li L, Shao N, Hu Z, Chen H, Xu L, et al. Triazine-modified dendrimer for efficient TRAIL gene therapy in osteosarcoma. Acta Biomaterialia. 2015. DOI: 10.1016/j.actbio.2015.01.007

[52] Akagi T, Baba M, Akashi M. Biodegradable nanoparticles as vaccine adjuvants and delivery systems: Regulation of immune responses by nanoparticle-based vaccine. Advances in Polymer Science. 2012. DOI: 10.1007/12_2011_150

[53] Barnier Quer C, Elsharkawy A, Romeijn S, Kros A, Jiskoot W. Cationic liposomes as adjuvants for influenza hemagglutinin: More than charge alone. European Journal of Pharmaceutics and Biopharmaceutics. 2012. DOI: 10.1016/j.ejpb.2012.03.013

[54] Kraft JC, Freeling JP, Wang Z, Ho RJY. Emerging research and clinical development trends of liposome and lipid nanoparticle drug delivery systems. Journal of Pharmaceutical Sciences. 2014. DOI: 10.1002/jps.23773

[55] Chen Y, Sun J, Lu Y, Tao C, Huang J, Zhang H, et al. Complexes containing cationic and anionic pH-sensitive liposomes: Comparative study of factors influencing plasmid DNA gene delivery to tumors. International Journal of Nanomedicine. 2013. DOI: 10.2147/IJN.S42800

[56] Li T, Takeoka S. A novel application of maleimide for advanced drug delivery: In vitro and in vivo evaluation of maleimide-modified pH-sensitive liposomes. International Journal of Nanomedicine. 2013. DOI: 10.2147/IJN.S47749

[57] Maitani Y, Igarashi S, Sato M, Hattori Y. Cationic liposome (DC-Chol/DOPE=1:2) and a modified ethanol injection method to prepare liposomes, increased gene expression. International Journal of Pharmaceutics. 2007. DOI: 10.1016/j.ijpharm.2007.04.035

[58] Puri A, Loomis K, Smith B, Lee J-H, Yavlovich A, Heldman E, et al. Lipid-based nanoparticles as pharmaceutical drug carriers: From concepts to clinic. Critical Reviews™ in Therapeutic Drug Carrier Systems. 2009. DOI: 10.1615/CritRevTherDrugCarrierSyst.v26.i6.10

[59] Korsholm KS, Hansen J, Karlsen K, Filskov J, Mikkelsen M, Lindenstrøm T, et al. Induction of CD8+ T-cell responses against subunit antigens by the novel cationic liposomal CAF09 adjuvant. Vaccine. 2014. DOI: 10.1016/j.vaccine.2014.05.050

[60] Wasungu L, Hoekstra D. Cationic lipids, lipoplexes and intracellular delivery of genes. Journal of Controlled Release. 2006. DOI: 10.1016/j.jconrel.2006.06.024

[61] Namvar A, Bolhassani A, Khairkhah N, Motevalli F. Physicochemical properties of polymers: An important system to overcome the cell barriers in gene transfection. Biopolymers. 2015. DOI: 10.1002/bip.22638

[62] Montenegro Stamford CT, Montenegro Stamford-Arnaud T, de Medeiros Cavalcante HM, Macedo RO, de Campos-Takaki M. Microbiological chitosan: Potential application as anticariogenic agent. Practical

Applications in Biomedical Engineering. 2012. DOI: 10.5772/54453

[63] Malhotra M, Tomaro-Duchesneau C, Saha S, Prakash S. Systemic siRNA delivery via peptide-tagged polymeric nanoparticles, targeting PLK1 gene in a mouse xenograft model of colorectal cancer. International Journal of Biomaterials. 2013. DOI: 10.1155/2013/252531

[64] Mumper RJ, Wang J, Claspell JM, Rolland AP. Novel polymeric condensing carriers for gene delivery. Proceedings of the Controlled Release Society. 1995;**22**:178-179

[65] Momenzadeh S, Sadeghi A, Vatandoust N, Salehi R. Evaluation of in vivo transfection efficiency of eudragit coated nanoparticles of chitosan-DNA: A pH-sensitive system prepared for oral DNA delivery. Iranian Red Crescent Medical Journal. 2015. DOI: 10.5812/ircmj.17(4)2015.16761

[66] Gao S, Hein S, Dagnæs-Hansen F, Weyer K, Yang C, Nielsen R, et al. Megalin-mediated specific uptake of chitosan/siRNA nanoparticles in mouse kidney proximal tubule epithelial cells enables AQP1 gene silencing. Theranostics. 2014. DOI: 10.7150/thno.7866

[67] Csaba N, Köping-Höggård M, Fernandez-Megia E, Novoa-Carballal R, Riguera R, Alonso MJ. Ionically crosslinked chitosan nanoparticles as gene delivery systems: Effect of PEGylation degree on in vitro and in vivo gene transfer. Journal of Biomedical Nanotechnology. 2009. DOI: 10.1166/jbn.2009.1017

[68] Yan C, Jie L, Yongqi W, Weiming X, Juqun X, Yanbing D, et al. Delivery of human NKG2D-IL-15 fusion gene by chitosan nanoparticles to enhance antitumor immunity. Biochemical and Biophysical Research Communications. 2015. DOI: 10.1016/j.bbrc.2015.05.065

[69] Lv H, Zhang S, Wang B, Cui S, Yan J. Toxicity of cationic lipids and cationic polymers in gene delivery. Journal of Controlled Release. 2006. DOI: 10.1016/j.jconrel.2006.04.014

[70] Matsumoto M, Kishikawa R, Kurosaki T, Nakagawa H, Ichikawa N, Hamamoto T, et al. Hybrid vector including polyethylenimine and cationic lipid, DOTMA, for gene delivery. International Journal of Pharmaceutics. 2008. DOI: 10.1016/j.ijpharm.2008.07.010

[71] Gulce Iz S, Inevi MA, Metiner PS, Tamis DA, Kisbet N. A BioDesign approach to obtain high yields of biosimilars by anti-apoptotic cell engineering: A case study to increase the production yield of anti-TNF alpha producing recombinant CHO cells. Applied Biochemistry and Biotechnology. 2018. DOI: 10.1007/s12010-017-2540-2

[72] Bivas-Benita M, Romeijn S, Junginger HE, Borchard G. PLGA-PEI nanoparticles for gene delivery to pulmonary epithelium. European Journal of Pharmaceutics and Biopharmaceutics. 2004. DOI: 10.1016/j.ejpb.2004.03.008

[73] Chumakova OV, Liopo AV, Andreev VG, Cicenaite I, Evers BM, Chakrabarty S, et al. Composition of PLGA and PEI/DNA nanoparticles improves ultrasound-mediated gene delivery in solid tumors in vivo. Cancer Letters. 2008. DOI: 10.1016/j.canlet.2007.11.023

[74] Ma YF, Yang YW. Delivery of DNA-based cancer vaccine with polyethylenimine. European Journal of Pharmaceutical Sciences. 2010. DOI: 10.1016/j.ejps.2010.02.009

[75] Liu X, Rocchi P, Peng L. Dendrimers as non-viral vectors for siRNA delivery. New Journal of Chemistry. 2012. DOI: 10.1039/c1nj20408d

[76] Liu C, Liu X, Rocchi P, Qu F, Iovanna JL, Peng L.

Arginine-terminated generation 4 PAMAM dendrimer as an effective nanovector for functional siRNA delivery in vitro and in vivo. Bioconjugate Chemistry. 2014. DOI: 10.1021/bc4005156

[77] Kang L, Gao Z, Huang W, Jin M, Wang Q. Nanocarrier-mediated co-delivery of chemotherapeutic drugs and gene agents for cancer treatment. Acta Pharmaceutica Sinica B. 2015. DOI: 10.1016/j.apsb.2015.03.001

[78] Kesharwani P, Iyer AK. Recent advances in dendrimer-based nanovectors for tumor-targeted drug and gene delivery. Drug Discovery Today. 2015. DOI: 10.1016/j.drudis.2014.12.012

[79] Dutta T, Garg M, Jain NK. Poly(propyleneimine) dendrimer and dendrosome mediated genetic immunization against hepatitis B. Vaccine. 2008. DOI: 10.1016/j.vaccine.2008.04.058

[80] Jilek S, Zurkaulen H, Pavlovic J, Merkle HP, Walter E. Transfection of a mouse dendritic cell line by plasmid DNA-loaded PLGA microparticles in vitro. European Journal of Pharmaceutics and Biopharmaceutics. 2004. DOI: 10.1016/j.ejpb.2004.03.038

[81] Kanazawa T, Takashima Y, Murakoshi M, Nakai Y, Okada H. Enhancement of gene transfection into human dendritic cells using cationic PLGA nanospheres with a synthesized nuclear localization signal. International Journal of Pharmaceutics. 2009. DOI: 10.1016/j.ijpharm.2009.06.015

[82] Bandyopadhyay A, Fine RL, Demento S, Bockenstedt LK, Fahmy TM. The impact of nanoparticle ligand density on dendritic-cell targeted vaccines. Biomaterials. 2011. DOI: 10.1016/j.biomaterials.2010.12.054

[83] Hamdy S, Haddadi A, Hung RW, Lavasanifar A. Targeting dendritic cells with nano-particulate PLGA cancer vaccine formulations. Advanced Drug Delivery Reviews. 2011. DOI: 10.1016/j.addr.2011.05.021

[84] Das J, Das S, Paul A, Samadder A, Bhattacharyya SS, Khuda-Bukhsh AR. Assessment of drug delivery and anticancer potentials of nanoparticles-loaded siRNA targeting STAT3 in lung cancer, in vitro and in vivo. Toxicology Letters. 2014. DOI: 10.1016/j.toxlet.2014.01.009

[85] Ediriwickrema A, Zhou J, Deng Y, Saltzman WM. Multi-layered nanoparticles for combination gene and drug delivery to tumors. Biomaterials. 2014. DOI: 10.1016/j.biomaterials.2014.07.043

[86] Tang X, Liang Y, Feng X, Zhang R, Jin X, Sun L. Co-delivery of docetaxel and Poloxamer 235 by PLGA-TPGS nanoparticles for breast cancer treatment. Materials Science and Engineering: C. 2015. DOI: 10.1016/j.msec.2015.01.033

[87] Blum JS, Saltzman WM. High loading efficiency and tunable release of plasmid DNA encapsulated in submicron particles fabricated from PLGA conjugated with poly-L-lysine. Journal of Controlled Release. 2008. DOI: 10.1016/j.jconrel.2008.04.002

[88] Díez S, Miguéliz I, De Ilarduya CT. Targeted cationic poly(D,L-lactic-co-glycolic acid) nanoparticles for gene delivery to cultured cells. Cellular & Molecular Biology Letters. 2009. DOI: 10.2478/s11658-009-0003-7

[89] Casettari L, Vllasaliu D, Castagnino E, Stolnik S, Howdle S, Illum L. PEGylated chitosan derivatives: Synthesis, characterizations and pharmaceutical applications. Progress in Polymer Science. 2012. DOI: 10.1016/j.progpolymsci.2011.10.001

[90] Betancourt T, Byrne JD, Sunaryo N, Crowder SW, Kadapakkam M, Patel S,

et al. PEGylation strategies for active targeting of PLA/PLGA nanoparticles. Journal of Biomedical Materials Research: Part A. 2009. DOI: 10.1002/jbm.a.32247

[91] Akgöl S, Kaçar Y, Özkara S, Yavuz H, Denizli A, Arica MY. Immobilization of catalase via adsorption onto L-histidine grafted functional pHEMA based membrane. Journal of Molecular Catalysis B: Enzymatic. 2001. DOI: 10.1016/S1381-1177(01)00029-7

[92] Hoffman AS. Hydrogels for biomedical applications. Advanced Drug Delivery Reviews. 2012. DOI: 10.1016/j.addr.2012.09.010

[93] Ma X, Wang H, Jin S, Wu Y, Liang XJ. Construction of paclitaxel-loaded poly(2-hydroxyethyl methacrylate)-g-poly(lactide)-1,2-dipalmitoyl-sn-glycero-3-phosphoethanolamine copolymer nanoparticle delivery system and evaluation of its anticancer activity. International Journal of Nanomedicine. 2012. DOI: 10.2147/IJN.S29371

[94] Tomar N, Tomar M, Gulati N, Nagaich U. pHEMA hydrogels: Devices for ocular drug delivery. International Journal of Health & Allied Sciences. 2012. DOI: 10.4103/2278-344X.107844

[95] Türkcan C, Akgöl S, Denizli A. Silanized polymeric nanoparticles for DNA isolation. Materials Science and Engineering: C. 2013. DOI: 10.1016/j.msec.2013.05.015

[96] Toprak A, Görgün C, Kuru CI, Türkcan C, Uygun M, Akgöl S. Boronate affinity nanoparticles for RNA isolation. Materials Science and Engineering: C. 2015. DOI: 10.1016/j.msec.2014.11.033

[97] Çimen D, Yilmaz F, Perçin I, Türkmen D, Denizli A. Dye affinity cryogels for plasmid DNA purification. Materials Science and Engineering: C. 2015. DOI: 10.1016/j.msec.2015.06.041

[98] Saglam-Metiner P. Development of high cationic nanotechnological adjuvant systems and demonstration of their efficiency in Her2 breast cancer DNA vaccine model [master's thesis]. 2017 (unpublished data)

[99] Samsonova O, Glinca S, Biela A, Pfeiffer C, Dayyoub E, Sahin D, et al. The use of isothermal titration calorimetry and molecular dynamics to show variability in DNA transfection performance. Acta Biomaterialia. 2013. DOI: 10.1016/j.actbio.2012.10.006

[100] Wang W, Nan W, Sun L, Liu W. A systemic gene vector constructed by zwitterionic polymer modified low molecular weight PEI. Reactive and Functional Polymers. 2013. DOI: 10.1016/j.reactfunctpolym.2013.05.003

[101] Hujaya SD, Marchioli G, Roelofs K, Van Apeldoorn AA, Moroni L, Karperien M, et al. Poly(amido amine)-based multilayered thin films on 2D and 3D supports for surface-mediated cell transfection. Journal of Controlled Release. 2015. DOI: 10.1016/j.jconrel.2015.01.034

[102] Koloskova OO, Gileva AM, Drozdova MG, Grechihina MV, Suzina NE, Budanova UA, et al. Effect of lipopeptide structure on gene delivery system properties: Evaluation in 2D and 3D in vitro models. Colloids Surfaces B Biointerfaces. 2018. DOI: 10.1016/j.colsurfb.2018.04.003

[103] Suschak JJ, Williams JA, Schmaljohn CS. Advancements in DNA vaccine vectors, non-mechanical delivery methods, and molecular adjuvants to increase immunogenicity. Human Vaccines & Immunotherapeutics. 2017. DOI: 10.1080/21645515.2017.1330236

[104] Donnelly JJ, Liu MA, Ulmer JB. Antigen presentation and DNA vaccines. American Journal of Respiratory and Critical Care Medicine. 2000

[105] Li L, Petrovsky N. Molecular mechanisms for enhanced DNA vaccine immunogenicity. Expert Review of Vaccines. 2016;**15**(3):313-329. DOI: 10.1586/14760584.2016.1124762

[106] Kim TW, Hung CF, Ling M, Juang J, He L, Hardwick JM, et al. Enhancing DNA vaccine potency by coadministration of DNA encoding antiapoptotic proteins. The Journal of Clinical Investigation. 2003. DOI: 10.1172/JCI200317293

[107] Leitner WW, Restifo NP. DNA vaccines and apoptosis: To kill or not to kill? The Journal of Clinical Investigation. 2003. DOI: 10.1172/JCI200319069

[108] Huang B, Mao CP, Peng S, He L, Hung CF, Wu TC. Intradermal administration of DNA vaccines combining a strategy to bypass antigen processing with a strategy to prolong dendritic cell survival enhances DNA vaccine potency. Vaccine. 2007. DOI: 10.1016/j.vaccine.2007.08.036

[109] Iz SG, Çalimlioğlu B, Gürhan SID. Using Bcl-xL anti-apoptotic protein for altering target cell apoptosis. Electronic Journal of Biotechnology. 2012. DOI: 10.2225/vol15-issue5-fulltext-2

Chapter 8

Role of Aryl Hydrocarbon-Ligands in the Regulation of Autoimmunity

Hana'a Burezq

Abstract

The aim of this study is to show the effects of activating aryl hydrocarbon receptor (AhR) by specific ligands, on the expression of responsive genes. Specific AhR-ligands were reported to play an important role in immune regulation. This chapter will focus mostly on the effects of activating AhR with different ligands on autoimmunity. Findings showed the possibility of using the AhR to treat inflammatory and autoimmune diseases in mice. AhR ligation with specific ligands can affect T cell differentiation, through activation of $CD4^{+}Foxp3^{+}$ regulatory T cells and downregulation of the pro-inflammatory T helper 17 cells. The results showed the effects of specific AhR-ligands on the production of pro-inflammatory and/or anti-inflammatory T cell subsets, the potential to use AhR-ligands in regulating the inflammation of organ/tissues in various diseases, suggesting that specific AhR-ligands could be used for immune regulation in pathogenesis of autoimmune diseases of human and mice.

Keywords: aryl hydrocarbon receptor, T helper 17, T regulatory cells, autoimmune disease, immune regulation

1. Introduction

The aryl hydrocarbon receptor (AhR) is a ligand-dependent transcription factor that mediates a variety of cellular events in many tissues [1]. AhR expression was found in many vertebrates such as rats and mice including fish. Therefore, it was suggested that AhR has a widespread biological function in animals, but its physiological role is not yet fully known. When AhR binds to xenobiotic ligands, the AhR regulates the expression of many genes including those encoding for cytochrome P450 enzymes. The activation of AhR was linked to variations in cell proliferation, apoptosis, tumor promotion, immune function, development, and reproductive functions [1, 2]. Many studies reported that the phenotype of AhR-deficient mice points to possible physiological functions of the receptor in liver, heart, ovary, vascular, and immune systems [2, 3]. The signaling pathway of AhR starts when AhR-ligand enters the responsive cell and binds with high affinity to the cytosolic AhR. The receptor exists as a multi-protein complex, containing two molecules of the chaperone heat shock protein of 90 kDa, the X-associated protein-2, and a 23-kDa co-chaperone protein [4]. The AhR undergoes conformational changes exposing a specific nuclear localization sequence which results in the translocation of the complex into the nucleus [5]. The ligand:AhR will then be released from this complex and bind to a related nuclear protein called AhR nuclear translocator (ARNT), which converts the AhR into its high-affinity DNA-binding form [6]. The ligand:AhR:ARNT complex binds to its specific DNA recognition site, the dioxin response elements (DREs), resulting in stimulation of the transcription of cytochrome P450 (CYP1A1) and other AhR-responsive genes. Once the AhR-ligand binds to its receptor, the AhR:ligand complex will translocate into the nucleus. The ligand:AhR will then be released from this complex and bind to ARNT, which converts the AhR into its high-affinity DNA-binding form, and then the ligand:AhR:ARNT complex will bind to the DRE, and as a result, transcription of cytochrome P450 and other AhR-responsive genes will start.

The present chapter highlights the effects of some AhR-ligands both exogenous and endogenous, on the secretion of pro- and/or anti-inflammatory cytokines which control the production of different T helper cell subsets, and consequently affects inflammation, and autoimmunity.

2. Categories of AhR-ligands

There are two major categories of AhR-ligands: exogenous and endogenous ligands. Exogenous ligands are those that are synthetic (formed as a result of non-biological activity) and/or naturally occurring dietary AhR-ligands. Endogenous ligands are those formed in biological systems as a result of natural processes in the body [7].

2.1 Exogenous AhR-ligands

2.1.1 Synthetic AhR-ligands

The synthetic AhR-ligands are in general high-affinity ligands and include halogenated aromatic hydrocarbons (HAHs) such as poly-halogenated dibenzo-*p*-dioxins. Synthetic ligands include also polycyclic aromatic hydrocarbons (PAHs) such as benzathracenes and related compounds [8]. HAHs represent the most potent type of AhR-ligands, with binding affinities in the pM to nM range. In contrast, PAHs bind to the AhR with lower affinity in the nM to μM range. The dioxin 2,3,7,8-tetrachlorodibenzo-*p*-dioxin (TCDD), which is a member of the HAH group, is considered as one of the most potent AhR agonists known. The potency of TCDD is about 1000-fold greater than that of PAH compounds [9]. It was observed that aryl hydrocarbon receptor-deficient mice, loss of responsiveness to TCDD and related chemicals [10]. Many genes are regulated by the AhR, especially those encoding xenobiotic metabolizing enzymes, such as cyp1a1. The induction of cyp1a1 is AhR-dependent response that has been observed in most species [11].

The physiological role of the AhR remains a key question, and to date no high-affinity endogenous ligand has been identified. The detailed analysis of AhR-ligand binding has mainly focused on the structurally related HAHs and PAHs. However, recent studies have demonstrated the ability of a structurally diverse range of chemicals to bind and/or activate AhR-dependent gene expression [12, 13].

These results suggest that AhR has a ligand-binding site with special characteristics. The identification and characterization of variety of naturally occurring AhR-ligands has started to redefine our ideas as to the structural specificity of AhR-ligand binding.

2.1.2 Naturally occurring dietary AhR-ligands

The major source of exposure of animals and humans to AhR-ligands both synthetic and natural comes from the diet. A number of studies have described and characterized a variety of naturally occurring dietary chemicals that can directly activate and/or inhibit the AhR signaling pathway. Many studies have documented a variety of naturally occurring dietary chemicals that can act as agonist/antagonist to AhR. It was reported that extracts of vegetables or vegetable-derived materials could induce CYP1A1 activity, the hallmark of AhR activation [14]. The ability of several dietary plant compounds, including 7,8-dihydrorutacarpine, indole 3-carbinol (I3C), indolo [3,2-b]carbazole (ICZ), dibenzoylmethanes, curcumin, quercetin, carotinoids (e.g., canthaxanthin and astaxanthin), pro-carotinoid, and β-apo-8'carotenal, to competitively bind to the AhR and stimulate AhR-dependent gene expression was also reported [15, 16]. Flavonoids are the largest group of naturally occurring dietary AhR-ligands which include flavones, flavanols, flavanones, and isoflavones. Flavonoids are found in dietary vegetables, fruits, and teas. These chemicals have strong antioxidative activity, anticarcinogenicity, and the ability to inhibit several enzymes such as protein kinases and cytochrome P450 [10, 17]).

Quercetin (3, 3′4′,5,7-pentahydroxy flavonol) is an AhR-ligand which could have both agonist and antagonist activity to AhR depending on the cell context and the experimental conditions [10]. The continuous administration of quercetin following TCDD exposure in C57Bl/6J mice prevented the reduction in body weight due to dioxin exposure [18], and quercetin treatment for 30 days was found to reduce hepatomegaly. Moreover, treating endothelial cells with 100-μM quercetin, following the treatment with the AhR-ligand polychlorinated biphenyls, was found to significantly reduce cyp1a1 mRNA level [19]. In addition to the ability of flavonoids to interact with the AhR, many of these flavonoids are also substrates of the CYP1A1 enzyme [20]. Flavonoid levels in human blood are usually in the μM concentration range, and this amount was reported to be sufficient to either inhibit or activate the AhR [21]. These findings suggest that quercetin could antagonize AhR causing significant suppression in the production of cyp1a1.

Curcumin [1,7-bis(4-hydrosy-3-methoxyphenyl)-1,6-hepta-diene-3,5-dione] is a naturally occurring dietary ligand of AhR. It is the main component (70–75%) of turmeric herb (*Curcuma longa*). Curcumin has a powerful anti-inflammatory, antioxidant, and antimicrobial activities [22, 23]. It has this ability because it can act through many cellular pathways including many transcription factors, hormones, growth factors, and their associated receptors. Also, curcumin is a powerful antitumor agent, due to its ability to dissociate the AhR/ARNT complex inside the nucleus [24]. The administration of curcumin suppresses cyp1a1 and 1b1 mRNA, induced by TCDD treatment. TCDD was reported to enhance AhR/ARNT-mediated cyp1a1 induction, and the expression of indoleamine-2,3-dioxygenase (IDO), which could enhance malignant transformation. In contrast, curcumin was observed to attenuate AhR/ARNT-mediated CYP induction by TCDD; thus, this mode of action may be the reason why curcumin could prevent malignant transformation, suggesting that curcumin could be used as a chemo-preventive or anticancer agent.

Thus, plant-derived materials and extracts contain AhR-ligands or products that can promptly be converted into AhR-ligands. They are perhaps the largest class of natural AhR-ligands to which humans and animals are exposed. These chemicals are capable of binding to AhR as ligands, and suppress the transformation of the receptor by simply inhibiting the phosphorylation of AhR and Arnt, by protein kinase C, which is responsible for this process.

2.2 Endogenous ligand/indoles

Recent studies reported that exposing tissue culture media to UV light enhances the induction of AhR-hydroxylase, an enzymatic activity usually associated with CYP1A1 requiring tryptophan for this response [25]. Many studies showed the ability of UV light to induce CYP1A1 in the skin and liver of rats and mice [26], suggesting that a diffusible AhR-ligand was generated in the skin. Thus, FICZ and other photooxidation products of tryptophan may actually be novel chemical messengers of light [25]. The ability of other endogenous indoles and indole metabolites to bind to the AhR has also been reported [27]. These studies demonstrated that tryptophan and naturally occurring tryptophan metabolites (tryptamine and indole acetic acid) can bind to and activate the AhR and AhR-dependent gene expression in both yeast and mammalian cells in culture. Tryptamine was also shown to be a relatively potent competitive inhibitor of CYP1A1-dependent enzymatic activity, suggesting that it may be a substrate for this enzyme [28]. More recently, it was observed that kyneurinine, additional metabolic breakdown products of tryptophan, could activate the AhR signaling pathway [29]. Because these chemicals are relatively weak ligands and only found at low concentration in cells, they are likely not endogenous activators in normal physiological conditions. However, if cellular concentrations of some tryptophan metabolites (i.e., tryptamine) are significantly elevated to 700 nM, for example, in this case, these ligands could activate the AhR receptor [30]. The solar spectrum is composed of various wavelength radiations having specific effects on skin. UV with the wave length between 295 and 215 nm is responsible for most sunburn and DNA damage. UV with the wavelength 315–400 nm could cause immune suppression. The visible light with the wavelength 400–700 nm was reported to enhance the production of reactive oxygen species and cause damage to macromolecules, whereas infrared induces heat damage and also alters mitochondrial integrity in skin cells, resulting in the generation of reactive oxygen species. All the wavelengths in solar spectrum together contribute to skin aging and wrinkling [27]. These findings can change the way we think about skin aging. UV-B was recently shown to interact with AhR in a reaction involving the formation of a tryptophan-derived photoproduct (FICZ) [26, 29]. In other words, the free amino acid tryptophan in skin cell cytoplasm can act as a chromophore to absorb UV-B energy and the resulting photoproduct activates AhR signaling, suggesting that to achieve effective dermo-protection, AhR must be blocked to neutralize some adverse effects of environmental factors.

3. Cytokines controlling T helper 17 and T regulatory cells polarization

3.1 T helper 17 subset (Th17)

There are specific cytokines which are important for the differentiation of naïve T cells into the T helper 17 subset. IL-6 and TGF-β together are important for the development of this population [31]. The blockade of IL-6 through anti-IL-6 antibody was found to inhibit the development of Th17 cells [32]. Furthermore, the addition of IL-1β to culture medium was reported to enhance the development of the Th17 subset. IL-1 receptor knockout mice showed a significant defect in the Th17 population [33]. IL-1β was found to enhance expression of the transcription factors orphan nuclear receptor (ROR-γt) and interferon regulatory factor-4 (IRF-4), which are responsible for the development of the Th17 subset [34]. The Th17 subset could secrete a variety of cytokines including IL-17A, IL-17F, IL-21, and IL-22, which have a pathogenic effect in certain autoimmune mouse models [35].

Moreover, IL-23 which is secreted by antigen-presenting cells (APCs) after pathogen recognition is important for the maintenance of the Th17 population [31]. These data suggested that the Th17 subset is a very sensitive subset requiring specific cytokines for development and maintenance.

3.2 T regulatory subset (Treg)

The presence of IL-10 and TGF-β was reported to skew the development of naïve T cell toward the development of T regulatory cells (Treg) [36]. The main function of Treg is to suppress the immune response, and to inhibit the production of pro-inflammatory cytokines such as IL-2 and IFN-γ. The development of this population could be inhibited in the presence of IL-1β and IL-6 [37]. Treg cells are characterized by the expression of CD25 and the forkhead box p3 (Foxp3) transcription factor [38]. The decreased production of pro-inflammatory cytokines such as IL-6 and IL-1β could help in skewing the differentiation of naïve T cells toward the development of the Treg subset.

4. Role of Th17 in autoimmunity

In some cases, the immune system attacks our own tissues, causing autoimmunity. IL-17-producing cells play important roles in the development of different autoimmune diseases including rheumatoid arthritis (RA), an inflammation disorder which attacks the synovial joints and multiple sclerosis (MS), characterized by inflammation of the myelin sheath, resulting in de-myelination. It was reported that IL-17-knockout mice were protected against these autoimmune diseases [39]. In contrast, a high level of IL-17 was detected in the serum of patients with MS, RA, and systemic lupus erythematous (SLE). This suggests that Th17 cells expressing high levels of ROR-γt and IL-23R could be one of the causes of these diseases [40]. In addition, it was also reported that the Th17 subset increases the severity of EAE, diabetes, and RA [41, 42].

5. Effects of AhR-ligands on the production of Th17/Treg subsets and autoimmunity

Differentiation of Th17 cells depends on the presence of interleukin (IL)-6 and transforming growth factor (TGF)-beta, and it could be regulated by the activation of AhR [43]. The differentiation of Th17 cells could be enhanced by endogenous AhR agonists found normally in culture medium. The RPMI culture medium could support very low levels of Th17 polarization, because it lacks the presence of these ligands. In contrast, Iscove's modified Dulbecco's medium (IMDM) is known to be rich in aromatic amino acids, such as tryptophan, histidine, and phenylalanine, that were thought to be the precursors of endogenous AhR-ligands and therefore significantly increase the development of Th17 cells [43]. In addition, treating naïve $CD4^{+}$T cells with the AhR-ligand FICZ in Th17 cell polarizing conditions helps in skewing the differentiation of naive $CD4^{+}$T cells, *in vitro*, toward the development of the Th17 population, and as a result, significant amounts of IL-17*a*, IL-17*f*, and IL-22 cytokines will be secreted. In contrast, a significant reduction in the development of Th17 cells was observed in AhR knockout mice, suggesting that the development of the Th17 cells was AhR dependent [35].

The activation of AhR with different AhR-ligands can regulate Treg/Th17 balance in mice. A significant increase in Treg population was noticed when AhR is activated with TCDD. In addition, suppression in the severity of EAE disease by a TGF-β1-dependent mechanism [44] was seen. Moreover, C57Bl/6J mice carrying the *d* allele of the Ahr gene (Ahr*d* mice) were characterized by a reduced affinity of about 10–100-fold for AhR-ligands due to a mutation in its ligand-binding site, and treating Ahr*d* mice with (1 μg/mouse) TCDD, had no significant effect on the severity of EAE and the development of Treg cells [44]. In contrast, when AhR binds to FICZ, the activation of the receptor will interfere with the differentiation of Treg development, and cause a significant induction of the Th17 subset and worsen EAE disease which suggests that AhR regulates Treg/Th17 subset differentiation in a ligand-specific manner [44]. These data suggested that different AhR-ligands have different effects on the production of pro- or anti-inflammatory T helper cell subsets, by controlling the production of different cytokines in the surrounding environment.

6. Effects of I3C and indirubin on immunoregulation

Indole-3-carbinol (I3C) (AhR-ligand) is found in cruciferous vegetables. Indirubin (IO) is another AhR-ligand, and is one of the components of the traditional Chinese medicine Danggui Longhui Wan. Although both of them are AhR-ligands, neither of these compounds bind the AhR as potently as TCDD. I3C and IO have anticancer properties, because they could inhibit cyclin dependent kinases that leads to cell cycle arrest in various cell lines. Moreover, both AhR-ligands were used to treat cancer. I3C has been used for the treatment of both breast and prostate cancer [45], while IO has been traditionally used for the treatment of chronic myelocytic leukemia [46]. I3C could downregulate the production of pro-inflammatory cytokines in macrophages [47, 48], whereas IO was reported to suppress these mediators in splenocytes and microglial cells [49].

A study was conducted to evaluate the effects of I3C and IO on specific immune cell populations, such as murine bone marrow-derived DCs, and the effect of these AhR-ligands was tested *in vivo*. The results showed that I3C and IO have immunosuppressive effects on DCs, which could promote a regulatory environment, thus could be useful to suppress chronic inflammatory diseases and/or autoimmunity *in vivo*. In addition, activating DC with lipopolysaccharide (LPS), after treating the cells with both AhR-ligands, suppresses the production of pro-inflammatory mediators including tumor necrosis factor-α (TNF-α), IL-1β, IL-6, IL-12, and nitric oxide but increased IL-10 levels. The DC treated with AhR-ligands was reported to upregulate some immune-regulating genes such as ALDH1A, IDO, and TGFB [50].

Both AhR-ligands were reported to suppress the levels of nuclear factor-kappa B (NF-κB), but only I3C suppressed the LPS-induced activity of RelB transcription factor encoded by the RELB gene. Finally, when naïve T cells were cultured with DCs treated with AhR-ligands, the increased production of $CD4^+Foxp3^+$ (Treg cells) [50] was seen.

The above observations suggest that I3C and IO have immunosuppressive and anti-inflammatory effects on DCs. Since these ligands are significantly less toxic than TCDD, these natural products may become useful therapeutics for the treatment of autoimmune and inflammatory diseases [50].

7. Effects of curcumin on Treg/Th17 balance and autoimmunity

The protective effect of curcumin was evaluated using ovalbumin (OVA)-induced allergic inflammation in mouse model of allergic asthma. This mouse model was established by ovalbumin. Mice were treated with different doses of curcumin (50, 100, and 200 mg/kg), and then the level of Treg/Th17-secreted cytokines was measured by enzyme-linked immunosorbent assay (ELISA). In addition, the percentages of Treg and Th17 were measured using flow cytometry assay. Results showed that curcumin caused a significant suppression in the production of Th17 subsets, and the secretion of IL-17 cytokines. In contrast, the AhR-ligand curcumin significantly enhanced the production of $CD4^{+}CD25^{+}$ T cell subsets. These findings suggest that curcumin could be used as therapeutic agent for patients with allergic asthma, because of its ability to significantly affect Treg/Th17 balance [51].

Curcumin plays an important role in multiple sclerosis (MS) autoimmune disease. It is characterized by some pathophysiological features such as breaching of blood-brain barrier (BBB) and injury to axons and myelin sheaths. Th17 cells play an important role in the pathophysiological process of MS. Curcumin is well known as active anti-inflammatory and neuroprotective agent if used prophylactically. Curcumin could inhibit neuroinflammation through multiple mechanisms in MS. First, CNS antigens will be captured by DC, and then the antigen will be presented to T cells, which will help in initiating inflammatory response [52]. This action will be followed by the secretion of different pro-inflammatory cytokines and enhancement of production of Th17 cells in circulation. The blood-brain barrier (BBB) usually expresses IL-17R and IL-22R receptors and the expression of these receptors will bridge the gap between Th17 and BBB tight junction that results in the disruption of tight junctions. This action will enhance the transmigration of Th17 across the BBB followed by the enhanced secretion of granzyme-B which in turn is found to initiate the killing of neurons. In contrast, curcumin treatment was found to inhibit the production and expansion of Th17 subsets in circulation. In addition, curcumin was reported to increase the expression of ZO-1 protein, an important tight junction protein, suggesting that curcumin can reduce neuroinflammation in MS autoimmune disease [52].

8. Discussions

How might different AhR-ligands, all with the ability to stimulate AhR-dependant gene transcription and promote Th17 cell development, promote either concomitant increases in Treg cells and lessen autoimmunity, or suppress Treg cell development and increase autoimmune activation? The presumed main function of AhR-induced transcriptional responses is to induce cytochrome P450 (e.g., CYP1A1) for detoxification of the detected aryl hydrocarbon. Indeed, FICZ is rapidly metabolized in a CYP-mediated reaction, within 1–3 hours [53] with a corresponding drop in AhR activation [54]. Thus, a transient AhR activation, even though promoting Th17 development and expansion, may ultimately terminate and allow Treg populations to emerge and dominate. In contrast, sustained AhR signaling might promote Foxp3 suppression and conversion of Treg to Th17 and Th1 cells.

Dietary AhR-ligands have also been suggested to act in an antagonistic manner to TCDD-induced AhR activation [55]. Additionally, although curcumin is able to act as a substrate for CYP1A1-mediated catabolism, it could partially decrease the accumulation of CYP1A1 mRNA [55] and antagonize CYP1A1 activity [56]. Therefore, interference with full AhR function, or metabolism of the inducing AhR-ligand or other endogenous ligands may be important in determining whether AhR-ligands result in regulatory and/or effector T cell development. Alternatively, certain AhR-ligands may induce distinct gene expression profiles [57], some of them promoting Th17 at the expense of Treg and others allowing the emergence of Treg.

The activation of AhR in DCs by some ligands may increase tolerogenic mediators, such as IDO, which promote Treg development. In support of this mechanism,

IDO expression was found to be increased in DCs by TCDD or FICZ [38]. The conversion of Treg to Th17 and Th17 to Th1 profiles has been reported and reprogramming of subsets might be possible by additional cytokine provision, such as IL-23, IL-6, or removal of reinforcement factors, such as IL-23 or AhR-ligands [38]. The reported ability of IDO products (i.e., tryptophan metabolites) to suppress ROR-γt and induce Foxp3$^+$Treg cells [58] may indicate Th17 to Treg conversion, or shift to an IL-10-producing subset might result during exposure to some AhR-ligands. Since some AhR-ligand treatments lead to Th17 responses in the absence of Treg responses, allowing enhanced autoimmunity, this suggests that these ligands may be useful to promote antitumor immunity. It also raises the possibility that the anticancer effects of curcumin and quercetin may be due to their ability to promote potent effector T cell subsets in addition to suppressing some chronic inflammatory states. Another potentially beneficial use of AhR-ligands that have the ability to increase Treg populations is for the prevention or treatment of autoimmune diseases.

Experimental evidence has shown that flavonoids could be used to treat many diseases including cancer [59, 60]. The administration of curcumin was found to block the formation of lesions and tumors in C57Bl/6J mice after implanting murine melanoma B16F10 cells in their neck and brain. Furthermore, curcumin treatment was observed to significantly inhibit the proliferation of PC-3 prostate tumor cells.

The proposed mechanism for this effect of curcumin was its ability to significantly suppress NF-κB and AP-1 signaling pathways in tumor cells [61, 62]. Curcumin was given orally at concentrations in the micro-molar range; however, results showed that the concentration of curcumin was in the nano-molar range in the plasma [63, 64], due to the extensive metabolism of curcumin in the intestine and liver, which prevents the maintenance of high concentration of curcumin in the plasma and tissues after taking it orally [65, 66]. The curcumin is effective on the cancer cells at high concentration which is difficult to be maintained for several hours even in the gastrointestinal tract [63]. This suggests that the potential of using curcumin for cancer treatment is limited when given orally and the intraperitoneal injection may be more effective.

In contrast, other studies have shown that high concentrations of curcumin were found to enhance chromosome malformation in different cell lines. The curcumin could cause DNA damage both *in vivo* and *in vitro* and increase the incidence of thyroid gland follicular cell hyperplasia and carcinogenic activity in the small intestine [67–69]. This was proposed mainly due to its ability to increase the production of reactive oxygen species (ROS) [70]. Other studies have shown that curcumin has the ability to suppress cytochrome P450 enzyme, glutathione, S-transferase, and UDP-glucuronosyltransferase, causing toxicity due to the increased level of drugs in the plasma [71]. Although lower concentrations of curcumin could enhance antioxidant activity, high concentrations of curcumin have shown pro-oxidant effects [63, 72].

Similarly, quercetin is known as an antioxidant, anti-inflammatory, and antimicrobial compound at low doses [73, 74]. In contrast, quercetin can enhance the production of ROS at higher concentrations [75]. ROS production by quercetin was found to kill some cancer cells, and quercetin complexes with bioactive compounds and metal ions such as lanthanum was reported to have powerful cytotoxic and antitumor properties at a concentration in the range of 100–1000 mM and the exposure time of tumor cells was around 3 hours. A quercetin/lanthanum complex was found to have a genotoxic effect on human cervical carcinoma cells due to ROS production [76].

Conflict of interest

There is no conflict of interest in this study.

Author details

Hana'a Burezq
Kuwait Institute for Scientific Research, Shuwaikh, Kuwait

*Address all correspondence to: haborizq@kisr.edu.kw

References

[1] Denison MS, Nagy SR. Activation of the aryl hydrocarbon receptor by structurally diverse exogenous and endogenous chemicals. Annual Review of Pharmacology and Toxicology. 2003;**43**:309-334

[2] Chan CY, Kim PM, Winn LM. TCDD-induced homologous recombination: The role of the Ah receptor versus oxidative DNA damage. Mutation Research. 2004;**563**:71-79

[3] Benedict JC, Lin TM, Loeffler IK, Peterson RE, Flaws JA. Physiological role of the aryl hydrocarbon receptor in mouse ovary development. Toxicological Sciences. 2000;**56**:382-388

[4] Kazlauskas A, Poellinger L, Pongratz I. Evidence that the co-chaperone p23 regulates ligand responsiveness of the dioxin (aryl hydrocarbon) receptor. The Journal of Biological Chemistry. 1999;**274**:13519-13524

[5] Hord NG, Perdew GH. Physicochemical and immunocytochemical analysis of the aryl hydrocarbon receptor nuclear translocator: Characterization of two monoclonal antibodies to the aryl hydrocarbon receptor nuclear translocator. Molecular Pharmacology. 1994;**46**:618-626

[6] Hankinson O. The aryl hydrocarbon receptor complex. Annual Review of Pharmacology and Toxicology. 1995;**35**:307-340

[7] Chang CY, Puga A. Constitutive activation of the aromatic hydrocarbon receptor. Molecular and Cellular Biology. 1998;**18**:525-535

[8] Bjeldanes LF, Kim JY, Grose KR, Bartholomew JC, Bradfield CA. Aromatic hydrocarbon responsiveness-receptor agonists generated from indole-3-carbinol in vitro and in vivo: Comparisons with 2,3,7,8-tetrachlorodibenzo-*p*-dioxin. Proceedings of the National Academy of Sciences of the United States of America. 1991;**88**:9543-9547

[9] Poland A, Knutson JC. 2,3,7,8-Tetrachlorodibenzo-p-dioxin and related halogenated aromatic hydrocarbons: examination of the mechanism of toxicity. Annual Review of Pharmacology and Toxicology. 1982;**22**:517-554

[10] Van der Heiden E, Bechoux N, Muller M, Sergent T, Schneider YJ, Larondelle Y, et al. Food flavonoid aryl hydrocarbon receptor-mediated agonistic/antagonistic/synergic activities in human and rat reporter gene assays. Analytica Chimica Acta. 2009;**637**:337-345

[11] Denison MS, Seidel SD, Rogers WJ, Ziccardi M, Winter GM, Heath-Pagliuso S. Natural and synthetic ligands for the Ah receptor. In: Puga A, Wallace KB, editors. Molecular Biology Approaches to Toxicology. Philadelphia: Taylor & Francis; 1998. pp. 393-410

[12] Heath-Pagliuso S, Rogers WJ, Tullis K, Seidel SD, Cenijn PH, Brouwer A, et al. Activation of the Ah receptor by tryptophan and tryptophan metabolites. Biochemistry. 1998;**37**:11508-11515

[13] Denison MS, Heath-Pagliuso S. The Ah receptor: A regulator of the biochemical and toxicological actions of structurally diverse chemicals. Bulletin of Environmental Contamination and Toxicology. 1998;**61**:557-568

[14] Teraoka H, Dong W, Tsujimoto Y. Induction of cytochrome P450 1A is required for circulation failure and edema by 2,3,7,8-tetrachlorodibenzo-p-dioxin in zebrafish. Biochemical and Biophysical Research Communications. 2003;**304**:223-228

[15] MacDonald CJ, Ciolino HP, Yeh GC. Dibenzoylmethane modulates aryl hydrocarbon receptor function and expression of cytochromes P50 1A1, 1A2, and 1B1. Cancer Research. 2001;**61**:3919-3924

[16] Ho JN, Jun W, Choue R, Lee J. I3C and ICZ inhibit migration by suppressing the EMT process and FAK expression in breast cancer cells. Molecular Medicine Reports. 2013;**7**:384-388

[17] Majewska M, Skrzycki M, Podsiad M, Czeczot H. Evaluation of antioxidant potential of flavonoids: An in vitro study. Acta Poloniae Pharmaceutica. 2011;**68**:611-615

[18] Ciftci O, Ozdemir I. Protective effects of quercetin and chrysin against 2,3,7,8-tetrachlorodibenzo-p-dioxin (TCDD) induced oxidative stress, body wasting and altered cytokine productions in rats. Immunopharmacology and Immunotoxicology. 2011;**33**:504-508

[19] Ramadass P, Meerarani P, Toborek M, Robertson LW, Hennig B. Dietary flavonoids modulate PCB-induced oxidative stress, CYP1A1 induction, and AhR-DNA binding activity in vascular endothelial cells. Toxicological Sciences. 2003;**76**:212-219

[20] Doostdar H, Burke MD, Mayer RT. Bioflavonoids: Selective substrates and inhibitors for cytochrome P450 CYP1A and CYP1B1. Toxicology. 2000;**144**:31-38

[21] Amakura Y, Tsutsumi T, Nakamura M, Kitagawa H, Fujino J, Sasak K, et al. Preliminary screening of the inhibitory effect of food extracts on activation of the aryl hydrocarbon receptor induced by 2,3,7,8-tetrachlorodibenzo-p-dioxin. Biological & Pharmaceutical Bulletin. 2002;**25**:272-274

[22] Bandgar BP, Jalde SS, Korbad BL, Patil SA, Chavan HV, Kinkar SN, et al. Synthesis and antioxidant, cytotoxicity and antimicrobial activities of novel curcumin mimics. Journal of Enzyme Inhibition and Medicinal Chemistry. 2012;**27**:267-274

[23] Patwardhan RS, Checker R, Sharma D, Kohli V, Priyadarsini KI, Sandur SK. Dimethoxycurcumin, a metabolically stable analogue of curcumin, exhibits anti-inflammatory activities in murine and human lymphocytes. Biochemical Pharmacology. 2011;**82**:642-657

[24] Choi H, Chun YS, Shin YJ, Ye S, SK KMS, Park JW. Curcumin attenuates cytochrome P450 induction in response to 2,3,7,8-tetrachlorodibenzo-p-dioxin by ROS-dependently degrading AhR and ARNT. Cancer Science. 2008;**99**:2518-2524

[25] Oberg M, Bergander L, Hakansson H, Rannug U, Rannug A. Identification of the tryptophan photoproduct 6-formylindolo[3,2-b] carbazole, in cell culture medium, as a factor that controls the background aryl hydrocarbon receptor activity. Toxicological Sciences. 2005;**85**:935-943

[26] Abel J, Haarmann-Stemmann T. An introduction to the molecular basics of aryl hydrocarbon receptor biology. The Journal of Biological Chemistry. 2010;**391**:1235-1248

[27] Svobodova A, Vostalova J. Solar radiation induced skin damage: Review of protective and preventive options. International Journal of Radiation Biology. 2010;**86**:999-1030

[28] Rannug A, Fritsche E. The aryl hydrocarbon receptor and light. The Journal of Biological Chemistry. 2006;**387**:1149-1157

[29] Agostinis P, Garmyn M, Van Laethem A. The aryl hydrocarbon receptor: An illuminating effector of

the UVB response. Science's STKE. 2007;**2007**(403):pe49

[30] Katiyar SK, Matsui MS, Mukhtar H. Ultraviolet-B exposure of human skin induces cytochromes P450 1A1 and 1B1. Journal of Investigative Dermatology. 2000;**114**:328-333

[31] Kimura A, Kishimoto T. IL-6: Regulator of Treg/Th17 balance. European Journal of Immunology. 2010;**40**:1830-1835

[32] Zhou L, Lopes JE, Chong MM, Ivanov II, Min R, Victora GD, et al. TGF-beta-induced Foxp3 inhibits T(H)17 cell differentiation by antagonizing ROR-gammat function. Nature. 2008;**453**:236-240

[33] Sutton C, Brereton C, Keogh B, Mills KH, Lavelle EC. A crucial role for interleukin (IL)-1 in the induction of IL-17-producing T cells that mediate autoimmune encephalomyelitis. The Journal of Experimental Medicine. 2006;**203**:1685-1691

[34] Chung Y, Chang SH, Martinez GJ, Yang XO, Nurieva R, Kang HS, et al. Critical regulation of early Th17 cell differentiation by interleukin-1 signaling. Immunity. 2009;**30**:576-587

[35] Veldhoen M, Hirota K, Westendorf AM, Buer J, Dumoutier L, Renauld JC, et al. The aryl hydrocarbon receptor links TH17-cell-mediated autoimmunity to environmental toxins. Nature. 2008;**453**:106-109

[36] Chen W, Jin W, Hardegen N, Lei KJ, Li L, Marinos N, et al. Conversion of peripheral $CD4^+CD25^+$ naive T cells to $CD4^+CD25^+$ regulatory T cells by TGF-beta induction of transcription factor Foxp3. The Journal of Experimental Medicine. 2003;**198**:1875-1886

[37] Afzali B, Mitchell P, Lechler RI, John S, Lombardi G. Translational mini-review series on Th17 cells: Induction of interleukin-17 production by regulatory T cells. Clinical and Experimental Immunology. 2010;**159**:120-130

[38] Murphy KM, Stockinger B. Effector T cell plasticity: flexibility in the face of changing circumstances. Nature Immunology. 2010;**11**:674-680

[39] Fletcher JM, Lalor SJ, Sweeney CM, Tubridy N, Mills KH. T cells in multiple sclerosis and experimental autoimmune encephalomyelitis. Clinical and Experimental Immunology. 2010;**162**:1-11

[40] Harris TJ, Grosso JF, Yen HR, Xin H, Kortylewski M, Albesiano E, et al. Cutting edge: An in vivo requirement for STAT3 signaling in TH17 development and TH17-dependent autoimmunity. Journal of Immunology. 2007;**179**:4313-4317

[41] Ghazavi A, Mosayebi G. The mechanism of sesame oil in ameliorating experimental autoimmune encephalomyelitis in C57BL/6 mice. Phytotherapy Research. 2011;**26**:34-38

[42] Petermann F, Korn T. Cytokines and effector T cell subsets causing autoimmune CNS disease. FEBS Letters. 2011;**585**:3747-3757

[43] Veldhoen M, Hirota K, Christensen J, O'Garra A, Stockinger B. Natural agonists for aryl hydrocarbon receptor in culture medium are essential for optimal differentiation of Th17 T cells. Journal of Experimental Medicine. 2009;**206**:43-49

[44] Quintana FJ, Basso AS, Iglesias AH, Korn T, Farez MF, Bettelli E, et al. Control of T(reg) and T(H)17 cell differentiation by the aryl hydrocarbon receptor. Nature. 2008;**453**:65-71

[45] Weng JR, Tsai CH, Kulp SK, Chen CS. Indole-3-carbinol as a chemopreventive and anti-cancer agent. Cancer Letters. 2008;**262**:153-163

[46] Eisenbrand G, Hippe F, Jakobs S, Muehlbeyer S. Molecular mechanisms of indirubin and its derivatives: Novel anticancer molecules with their origin in traditional Chinese phytomedicine. Journal of Cancer Research and Clinical Oncology. 2004;**130**:627-635

[47] Chang HP, Wang ML, Hsu CY, Liu ME, Chan MH, Chen YH. Suppression of inflammation-associated factors by indole-3-carbinol in mice fed high-fat diets and in isolated, co-cultured macrophages and adipocytes. International Journal of Pediatric Obesity. 2011;**35**:1530-1538

[48] Tsai SA, Shameli J, Yamanouchi X, Clemente-Casares X, Wang J, Serra P, et al. Reversal of autoimmunity by boosting memory-like auto-regulatory T cells. Immunity. 2010;**32**:568-580

[49] Jung HJ, Nam KN, Son MS, Kang H, Hong JW, Kim JW, et al. Indirubin-3'-oxime inhibits inflammatory activation of rat brain microglia. Neuroscience Letters. 2011;**487**:139-143

[50] Benson JM, Shepherd DM. Dietary ligands of the aryl-hydrocarbon receptor induce anti-inflammatory and immunoregulatory effects on murine dendritic cells. Toxicological Sciences. 2011;**124**:327-338

[51] Chunhun MA, Zhanqiany MA, Qiang FU, Ma S. Curcumin attenuates allergic airway inflammation by regulation of CD4+CD25+ regulatory T cells (Treg)/Th17 balance in ovalbumin-sensitized mice. Fitoterapia. 2013;**87**:57-64

[52] Xie L, Li XK, Takahara S. Curcumin has bright prospects for the treatment of multiple sclerosis. International Immunopharmacology. 2011;(3):323-330

[53] Bergander L, Wincent E, Rannug A, Foroozesh M, Alworth W, Rannug U. Metabolic fate of the Ah receptor ligand 6-formylindolo[3,2-b]carbazole. Chemico-Biological Interactions. 2004;**149**:151-164

[54] Wei YD, Helleberg H, Rannug U, Rannug A. Rapid and transient induction of CYP1A1 gene expression in human cells by the tryptophan photoproduct 6-formylindolo[3,2-b] carbazole. Chemico-Biological Interactions. 1998;**110**:39-55

[55] Ciolino HP, Daschner PJ, Wang TT, Yeh GC. Effect of curcumin on the aryl hydrocarbon receptor and cytochrome P450 1A1 in MCF-7 human breast carcinoma cells. Biochemical Pharmacology. 1998;**56**:197-206

[56] Rinaldi AL, Morse MA, Fields HW, Rothas DA, Pei P, Rodrigo KA, et al. Curcumin activates the aryl hydrocarbon receptor yet significantly inhibits (−)-benzo(a)pyrene-7R-trans-7,8-dihydrodiol bioactivation in oral squamous cell carcinoma cells and oral mucosa. Cancer Research. 2002;**62**:5451-5456

[57] Ciolino HP, Daschner PJ, GC Y. Dietary flavonols quercetin and kaempferol are ligands of the aryl hydrocarbon receptor that affect CYP1A1 transcription differentially. Biochemical Journal. 1999;**340**:715-722

[58] De Luca A, Montagnoli C, Zelante TP, Bonifazi S, Bozza S, Moretti S, et al. Functional yet balanced reactivity to *Candida albicans* requires TRIF, MyD88, and IDO-dependent inhibition of Rorc. The Journal of Immunology. 2007;**179**:5999-6008

[59] Anand P, Sundaram C, Jhurani S, Kunnumakkara AB, Aggarwal BB. Curcumin and cancer: An "old-age" disease with an "age-old" solution. Cancer Letters. 2008;**267**:133-164

[60] Ravindran J, Prasad S, Aggarwal BB. Curcumin and cancer cells: how many ways can curry kill tumor

cells selectively? The AAPS Journal. 2009;**11**:495-510

[61] Langone P, Debata PR, Dolai S, Curcio GM, Inigo Jdel R, Raja K, et al. Coupling to a cancer cell-specific antibody potentiates tumoricidal properties of curcumin. International Journal of Cancer. 2011;**131**:E569-E578

[62] Liu S, Wang Z, Hu Z, Li K, Sun Z. Anti-tumor activity of curcumin against androgen-independent prostate cancer cells via inhibition of NF-κB and AP-1 pathway in vitro. Journal of Huazhong University of Science and Technology. Medical Sciences. 2011;**31**:530-535

[63] Lopez-Lazaro M. Anticancer and carcinogenic properties of curcumin: Considerations for its clinical development as a cancer chemopreventive and chemotherapeutic agent. Molecular Nutrition & Food Research. 2008;**52**:S103-S137

[64] Vareed SK, Kakarala M, Ruffin MT, Crowell JA, Normolle DP, Djuric Z, et al. Pharmacokinetics of curcumin conjugate metabolites in healthy human subjects. Cancer Epidemiology, Biomarkers & Prevention. 2008;**17**:1411-1417

[65] Ireson CR, Orr S, Jones DJ, Verschoyle R, Lim CK, Luo JL, et al. Characterization of metabolites of the chemopreventive agent curcumin in human and rat hepatocytes and in the rat in vivo, and evaluation of their ability to inhibit phorbol ester-induced prostaglandin E2 production. Cancer Research. 2001;**61**:1058-1064

[66] Ireson CR, Jones DJ, Orr S, Coughtrie MW, Boocock DJ, Williams ML, et al. Metabolism of the cancer chemopreventive agent curcumin in human and rat intestine. Cancer Epidemiology, Biomarkers & Prevention. 2002;**11**:105-111

[67] Cao J, Jia L, Zhou HM, Liu Y, Zhong LF. Mitochondrial and nuclear DNA damage induced by curcumin in human hepatoma G2 cells. Journal of Toxicological Sciences. 2006;**91**:476-483

[68] Dance-Barnes ST, Kock ND, Moore JE, Lin EY, Mosley LJ, D'Agostino RB, et al. Lung tumor promotion by curcumin. Carcinogenesis. 2009;**30**:1016-1023

[69] Verschoyle RD, Steward WP, Gescher AJ. Putative cancer chemopreventive agents of dietary origin—How safe are they? Nutrition and Cancer. 2007;**59**:152-162

[70] Aykin-Burns N, Ahmad IM, Zhu Y, Oberley LW, Spitz DR. Increased levels of superoxide and H_2O_2 mediate the differential susceptibility of cancer cells versus normal cells to glucose deprivation. Biochemical Journal. 2009;**418**:29-37

[71] Mancuso C, Barone E. Curcumin in clinical practice: Myth or reality? Trends in Pharmacological Sciences. 2009;**30**:333-334

[72] Sandur SK, Ichikawa H, Pandey MK, Kunnumakkara AB, Sung B, Sethi G, et al. Role of pro-oxidants and antioxidants in the anti-inflammatory and apoptotic effects of curcumin (diferuloylmethane). Free Radical Biology and Medicine. 2007;**43**:568-580

[73] Bischoff SC. Quercetin: Potentials in the prevention and therapy of disease. Current Opinion in Clinical Nutrition and Metabolic Care. 2008;**11**:733-740

[74] Mamani-Matsuda M, Rambert J, Malvy D, Lejoly-Boisseau H, Daulouède S, Thiolat D, et al. Quercetin induces apoptosis of *Trypanosoma brucei* gambiense and decreases the proinflammatory response of human macrophages. Antimicrobial Agents and Chemotherapy. 2004;**48**:924-929

[75] De Marchi U, Biasutto L, Garbisa S, Toninello A, Zoratti M. Quercetin can act either as an inhibitor or an inducer of the mitochondrial permeability transition pore: A demonstration of the ambivalent redox character of polyphenols. Biochimica et Biophysica Acta. 2009;**1787**:1425-1432

[76] Durgo K, Halec I, Sola I, Franekić J. Cytotoxic and genotoxic effects of the quercetin/lanthanum complex on human cervical carcinoma cells in vitro. Archives of Industrial Hygiene and Toxicology. 2011;**62**:221-227